FATBUSTERS

The fast fat-burning exercise programme

FATBUSTERS

The fast fat-burning exercise programme

Jamie Addicoat

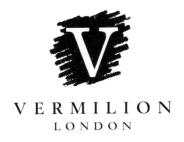

VERMILION
LONDON

Published in 1992 by Vermilion
an imprint of Ebury Press
Random Century House
20 Vauxhall Bridge Road
London SW1V 2SA

British Library Cataloguing-in-Publication Data

A catalogue record for this book is available from the
British Library

ISBN 0 09 175297 3

Edited by Susan Fleming
Designed by Jerry Goldie
Photography by Jon Stewart
Typeset in Memphis by Textype Typesetters, Cambridge
Printed and bound in Great Britain by the Bath Press,
Avon

A NOTE OF CAUTION

Before beginning this, or any other, exercise programme, it is advisable to obtain the
approval and recommendations of your doctor. While you are on this, or any,
exercise programme, it is advisable to visit your doctor for periodic monitoring.
Fatbusters is intended for people of all ages in good health.

CONTENTS

ACKNOWLEDGMENTS

First and foremost, I would like to thank my wife Jane and our daughter Billy Joe for their support during the tough times, but as they say, when the going gets tough, the tough get going. Thank you, John and Janet, my parents, plus Kathy and the rest of the Addicoat clan for the attitude that you have instilled (not to be mistaken for distilled) in me. A very special thanks to all the dudes out there who have done it 'The Addicoat Way' because without you there ain't no Fatbusters. Fatbusters of the world, stand up and be counted, it's your time.

No thanks to all the so-called fitness professionals and various other rip-off merchants who have never had a kind word for me or other teachers that don't fit into their little worlds. You're welcome to it.

A special thanks to Mambo, Converse and Pure Energy for supplying the only gear to be seen in on the street or in the class. Thanks to the Great British Press for giving me a great run for six years, cheers. A special thanks to Amelia Thorpe and Gillian Haslam at Ebury Press for treading where no man dared before, and letting the word be printed. To finish this movie off, thanks to all the dudes that have helped and survived all the effing and blinding over the years, especially the teachers with whom I teach, the dudes in the book, and the dudes that keep trucking on in the classes. Without you, it's just another story.

A FEW FLATTERIES . . .

'Jamie, "trainer to the superstars"'

Geena Davies

'Jamie, phitness was "ph-phun"'

Max Headroom

'Jamie – a million thanks for giving Mozart some muscle'

Tom Hulce

'Jamie is the bee's knees. Without him there would be no "Doing the Do"'

Betty Boo

'Jamie – a cruel genius'

Richard Jobson

'All ye of little faith – prepare to meet the ultimate workout'

John Lynch

'Jamie is the only man in my life who can crack the whip and get away with it'

Gina Bellman

'Jamie is the only straight person I'll let near me in the gym – I love pumping iron with Jamie'

Boy George

The Law According to Jamie

(Not quite the 10 Commandments, but nearly . . .)

1. The instructions and advice presented in this book are in no way intended as a substitute for medical guidance.

2. This programme is not suitable for men or women in any form of pregnancy.

3. If you suffer from high blood pressure, have a history of heart disease or any other imaginable disease known to man, consult your doctor before commencing an exercise programme.

4. Do not go past Go before doing your Fitness Testings. If any problems, consult with a qualified person before collecting £200.

5. Learn your Fatbusting training heart ranges first, because without them you ain't losing nothing.

6. No workouts without warming-up and cooling-down.

7. Remember, any pain – no train.

8. Remember your floor's probably not like mine, so always bend your knees on impact, and land toe to heel in any jogging movements.

9. It's not a fashion show, so wear comfortable loose clothing throughout. Sling out those Lycra numbers, and get real . . .
See you on the thin side!

INTRODUCTION

Once upon a time, in a far-off land, lived a scrawny nine-stone weakling (less of the weakling) called Jamie. One day he plucked up the courage to go to his local health club, and to his surprise and delight, he discovered something that was going to turn him from a skinny youth into a lean, mean fighting machine. He pumped iron until his eyes bulged, rode the bike until his legs ached, and did so many aerobic classes he had leotard burns on his thighs. What did he have to show for all this? Sweet nothing. Well, almost nothing. . . . He had gained three pounds. Jamie was now totally disillusioned with the whole health and fitness game, but being the kind of guy he was, he devoted the next two years to pondering the problems of the health and fitness lark, and finally found the solutions to everybody's problems.

At this point Jamie left his place of birth and travelled across the oceans (probably in chains) to bring the word to the masses. He started work at a very 'ex' well-known gym in Central London and started to work on his theories and test them. They came to a head after completing a stint of personal training with a very fat and unhappy advertising executive. The man whom we will call Man approached Jamie – yes, me – in a very depressed state after a nasty experience with 'black bombers' or appetite depressants. Apparently Man had been prescribed these tabs for weight loss, and to his joy the weight dropped off dramatically and very fast, but the side effects wasted his mind. After deciding to drop the drugs, the weight returned with a vengeance, faster and more than ever before, so he thought as a last resort exercise would be the answer.

So we started exercising, five days a week, controlling his eating and drinking, and lo and behold the weight started dropping off again. The other added bonus Man discovered was that he was getting fit again, a feeling he hadn't experienced in many years. Most of the time the feeling of well-being and being able to hold his own in the gym took precedence over the weight loss. We used cross-training theories well before they became the vogue. After finishing our stint Man thanked me, but left me these thoughts to ponder.

- Do you know what it's like to come into these palaces of thinness, and do things that the beautiful people take for granted, like showering, trying to buy training gear when you're a size 24 and the shops only stock size 16 max, attending classes when the teachers try to blank you because you're fat and unfit, and anyway the classes were all whooping and yelping and pretty dancey. . . .

So I thought it's time to start a class for the great unfit and fat and, in 1985, Fatbusters was born.

- **'Be master of your own nudity.'**
  In other words, not what the magazines, books, videos and so-called fitness gurus dictate you should be. Size 20 is as good as size 8.
- **'Enjoy the fitness game, so that you can maximise on your vices.'**
  Life as we know it shouldn't stop because you want to be fit again.

In the early days the class was real basic with very little music. These days the class has progressed with the times, slightly more dancified but not much, with a far greater range of exercises and small weights work, but still with all the screaming, hard work and fun. The class has always been hard, but I'm a firm believer in the deep end first, and the going can only get better. As I look around the fitness scene in Britain, I find that I see various aspects of Fatbusters in most classes that are of any value, and even all the basic concepts of cross-training I used in my class applied to gym workouts.

I've had them all through the classes over the years, the rich and famous, the extra, extra large and the not so large, the fit and unfit, the old and young and the ones along for the giggle, and apart from a few we've all had a good time, lost loads of weight and become real fit. We've had some amazing weight losses – 9 stone in one year Andy, 5 stone Jamie and Anne and others too numerous to name – but the biggest buzz I've had is the attitude these people have gained. For at the end of the day, attitude makes that little bit extra that you need to succeed. The exercise is right, get the mind right. It takes time, plenty of sweat, blood, guts and tears. Welcome to the original Fatbusters, a layman's guide to health and fitness!

Jamie 'Fatbusting' Addicoat, 1992

The Real Story: Before Fatbusters

6 I got up this morning, gazed into the mirror and wished that I was thin again. How many mornings have I done this? Pick up the morning rag, and have my optical senses assaulted by skinny little darlings, selling every magic potion and cure available to man, promising to cure my weight problem forever, only for a tenner. How many tenners will I spend before I learn?

Now on top of this, a new problem has emerged to throw my whole life into chaos. The 90s brought out all the do-gooders, saying you should be content with your body as it is: curves are back; we should be happy with our God-given shape. Everything is back to the 60s all of a sudden, peace and contentment, fat is beautiful .... Nonsense, being fat is not happy, fat people are unhappy people. Make your mind up, is it size 10 again or size 24 for this decade?

I'm only a poor brainwashed reader of the British Press being led down the garden path. Do I exercise, do I diet, do I swallow these pills, do I wait for that magic cure they keep promising, or do I stick my fingers up at it all and pretend I'm a happy little round one with metabolic problems? Help?

I've tried it all and lost a few pounds here and there. Everybody suggests I try exercise, but where am I going to find a class that isn't going to make me feel like slitting my throat every time I waddle into the room? They're all so intense, pitched at people who look like they run a marathon without breaking into a sweat, girls who look as though their only excess weight problem in life has been at the airport. My God, I hate it – rows and rows of scantily-clad gods paying homage to themselves. I think I'll crawl out and eat another chocolate bar. 9

WHAT IS FATBUSTERS?

Fatbusters is a force to be reckoned with, combining all aspects of fitness training with a healthy long-term eating plan. This no-nonsense class combines low-impact and high-impact exercise, weight training, circuit training and a real good time. The aim of Fatbusters is to increase your basic metabolic rate via low-intensity exercise, to improve your stamina, tone your body, burn fat effectively, and put the fun back into being fit. Exercise is always considered that little bit much for your average fattie, due to the fact they are generally considered too unfit to participate in any exercise regime for any great length of time. This just is not true. Just because you're fat doesn't mean you're an invalid. Without any degree of fitness – which is far more obtainable than radical body changes – forget any massive weight loss in the immediate future. The first part of any weight-loss programme should be geared to getting some base fitness and then watch the weight drop off. In all my experience with the overweight, the feeling of fitness and well-being takes precedence over the initial weight loss. This latter will come as your level of fitness gradually increases.

Fatbusters is not for the skinny, or the poseurs, or those who want to dance in lines. Those who can't cope with a little bit of good fun and smut with a load of aggro thrown in need read no further. Fatbusters is not a fleeting fitness fad, but is here to stay. Amen.

Why Do We Get Fat?

Genetics and upbringing play major parts in whether you are fat or will become fat. Two joe-average parents result in a 'pyjama goblin'* with a slight chance of being overweight. One fat oldie will result in a 40% chance of a fat child, and two fat parents may result in a possible 80% fat 'rug rat'*.   *Child.

But at the end of the day, fatness is down to two processes. One is hypertrophy, or the *enlargement* of existing fat cells, which can generally be put down to the fact that you're bone idle and eat too much. The other is hyperplasia, or an *increase* in fat cells, which can lead to an increase in fatness. In the dark dim past it was thought that fat cells were laid down in the formative stages of your life, and were not prone to change. However, we have since discovered that fat-cell numbers can be changed at three particular stages in life through bad eating and inactivity.

● Before your birth (seeing as you are confined during this stage of life, blame your Mum).
● In the early years (no more sweets, kiddies).
● Pre-puberty.

The bad news, dudes, is that once you've increased the fat cells there's no turning back, excepting in size of the cell (atrophy, or the reverse of hypertrophy). So roll on pre-natal exercises for the foetus, kiddies' aerobics and pre-puberty raves without the 'Es'.

Fat and calories

To put it simply, foods taken in above energy expended daily, results in you enlarging the size of your fat cells. If you eat more than you burn off daily, the fat piles on.

Anything you eat or drink, whether protein, carbohydrate, fat or alcohol, is measured in calories (or, more properly, units of 1000 calories, Kilocalories or Kcal). For instance, both 1 gram of protein and 1 gram of carbohydrate equal 4 calories, while 1 gram of fat equals 9 calories and 1 gram of alcohol about 7 calories. As fat is the form in which you store excess calories, anything that supplies the calories in *excess* is converted and stored as fat.

We all have different recommended daily calorie requirements: growing children of one and two years old need

The Pros and Cons of Being Fit According to Jamie

We instinctively assume that being fit is better than being unfit, when we all know that both fitness and unfitness have their advantages and disadvantages, as you're about to find out. **Welcome** to the health zone. Think hard and long before you make that first step either way.

Advantages of being fit
- You will live longer, unless of course you're waiting for major surgery on the NHS.
- Your teeth will last longer, and chew food far more efficiently.
- Odds on that you will be in a better mood 95% of the time, and at least 5% happier on 75% of the remaining 5% of the time.
- You will be able to recite and understand statistics.
- Your marriage will last longer, unless of course you're not married, when your one-night stands will be more fulfilling.
- You are 50% less likely to get stuck in supermarket turnstiles.
- Your spleen will survive on average five years more.
- You are likely to be able to drink 5% cheaper for 75% of 90% of your remaining years.
- You are less likely to be harpooned at the beach.
- You will be able to wear all the rage clothes, instead of citing the age-old excuse 'I think he's a bum designer anyway', when we all know that all that comes in size 22 is potato sacks.
- No more paying for two seats on public transport.

Advantages of being unfit

- You are better at holding down loose floorboards.
- You will absorb less radiation from microwaves and other radioactive things.
- You will be more effective at bribery, treason and at least a majority of all other major crimes.
- You will be far more capable of activities such as free-fall parachute jumping, deep-sea diving, kick-starting jumbo jets and any other activity that relies on the force of gravity working against body mass.
- You will be far more attractive to at least 60% of the larger, four-legged mammals.
- You will be offered loads of film work, like sinking in quicksand, the new marshmallow monster in Ghostbusters 3 etc.

So what can we gather from all this? It's not essential or even desirable to be fit to enjoy life. Plenty of opportunities exist for the great fat and unfit. At the end of the day it's up to you alone as to whether you think being fit is better than being unfit.

But if you do decide you have a fitness problem, and that being fit would suit your lifestyle, how do you tackle the problem? You have a choice of putting the blame on yourself (the manly thing to do), or putting the blame on somebody or something else (the sensible cowardly thing to do). If you decide to blame yourself then the answer lies in dated actions such as actress and starlet workouts, new gee-whiz diets and fad exercise regimes. But if you decide to put the blame elsewhere, you need to look around for a suitable disease to explain your great unfitness away. And in the words of that great poet of the screen, Sly Stallone, 'you're the disease and I'm the cure'.

The cure is Fatbusters – cross-training, new body workouts and healthy eating. So it's time to get real and be master of your own nudity.

1200–1400 calories daily, *more* than many calorie-controlled diets allow slimmers! A man who is very active could need food supplying over 3000 calories a day to keep him going.

How to determine your calorific needs

1. Desirable weight (lbs) × 10 = basal calories

2. Add activity calories:

- **Sedentary = desirable weight × 3**
- **Moderate = desirable weight × 5**
- **Active = desirable weight × 10**

3. If you want to lose weight, subtract calories for weight loss. A loss of some 500 calories per day will result in the loss of a pound (roughly 0.5 kg) per week.

The so-called standards of body-fat percentages for men and women, and how you can test for your own fat levels, are detailed on pages 47–9.

Controlling the fat

The average Western diet comprises 42% fat (of which 16% is saturated and 26% is poly- and monounsaturated), 12% proteins and 46% carbohydrates (of which 28% is complex carbs and 18% simple carbs). The ideal diet should be 30% fats, only 10% of it saturated, 12% proteins and 58% carbohydrates, of which only 10% should be simple.

To gain long-term results, any weight-control programme should take the following into account.

1. It should involve changes that can be maintained for life. Crash dieting slows the metabolic rate – the rate at which the body uses up fat – and this can lead to weight gain when the diet returns to normal.

2. It should aim for gradual weight loss coupled with exercise. This not only maintains the weight loss but increases the metabolic rate so that more calories are 'burnt' on a day-to-day basis. A 2–2¼ lb (roughly 1kg) weight loss per week is considered safe, healthy and effective. With a Fatbusting exercise programme, expect a bit more.

3. It should recognise that dieting simply treats the symptoms, not the *cause* of why you are over-eating. Find the cause and treat it.

Turn to page 139 for a brief outline of a healthy eating and reducing plan according to Jamie.

Why Exercise?

I think in this country, the number one reason why we exercise (or attempt to) is that it will improve our appearance. If the exercise is right, body shape, body tone and body fat can all be beneficially affected.

In very simple terms, an exercise uses both carbohydrate and fat for fuel. Generally speaking, short high bursts of exercise such as sprinting, squash etc, use carbohydrate as the fuel source. This sort of exercise is known as anaerobic (see page 21). Exercise which involves large groups of muscles but which is of longer duration also 'eats' carbohydrate, but uses fat as the primary fuel source. This is known as aerobic exercise. So, a workout based on aerobic exercise will help you lose fat. (This is all described in much greater detail on page 21.)

That's what Fatbusting will do for you from a cosmetic point of view, which is important for the majority of us. But, apart from making us sweat and stink, what else does all this working out do?

Regular exercise ensures important benefits to all of your physiological systems and psychological functioning. These other benefits may be less visible than improved shape and body tone, but they do contribute to the quality of your life. They reduce risks of illness and may even extend your lifespan (making promises again). Listed below are some of the major effects you can expect from the right kind of exercise regime performed regularly.

The heart

The average resting heart rate is approximately 72 beats per minute. Cardiovascular fitness-based activities strengthen the heart, helping to circulate more blood per beat, the result being a lower resting heart rate. A lower resting heart rate suggests that the cardiovascular – your heart and lungs – system is working far more efficiently.

Blood vessels

High blood pressure is the major factor involved in strokes. Regular exercise helps to make the blood vessels more elastic and less obstructed with fat, permitting freer circulation of blood and therefore lowering blood pressure.

The lungs

Cardiovascular exercises strengthen your lungs as well, enlarging their capacity to absorb oxygen and expel waste products.

A conditioned heart and lung system works efficiently to minimise the risks of heart disease. As the cardiovascular system adapts to more strenuous exercise, the heart rate actually returns to its resting level more quickly after exertion.

The metabolism

A fit individual actually burns off more calories, even while resting. This promotes leanness and helps reach and maintain ideal body fat percentages.

Body composition

A fitter body is a less fat body, because aerobic exercise uses up excess fat stores for energy. The result is a leaner frame with proportionately more muscle.

Your muscles

Unexercised muscles don't turn into fat, but they do atrophy and become weak. Only regular exercise makes the musculature strong, firm, defined and efficient.

Your bones and joints

Bones tend to become porous and brittle with age, but regular exercise helps make them more dense and resilient. It has been recognised in the last few years that exercises which apply force to bones (not directly, I might add, that's called a broken bone!) will help add to their density or maintain this density. People who exercise regularly, particularly those involved in weight-bearing activities, have far greater bone density than those on the other side of the fence. At present it's not known the amount of activity that is needed to bring about this change in bone density, but it is clear that calcium loss is proportionate to the level of your inactivity. (Oestrogen is also implicated in menopausal bone brittleness or osteosporosis.)

It seems that even the slightest bit of weight-bearing exercise will be beneficial at the end of the day, fitness also giving the joints a much wider range of motion which enables you to move more freely without discomfort. Maybe in future years, exercise and weight training will replace hip transplants etc for older people on the NHS.

Ageing

As for slowing down the marching of time, even though nothing has been proved conclusively, compare the older people who have exercised all their lives to their counterparts who have done sweet FA all their lives. Their lungs and heart are still going hell for leather generally, their minds are far more alert than their mates in the Zimmer frame, and they are less prone to osteosporosis. Fitness won't stop the wrinkles, and you will still make the grave like the rest of the world, but it will be a far more enjoyable trip then if you hadn't bothered.

Your mental functioning

As people become more dedicated to their exercise regimes, they also discover they've gained improved concentration and alertness without boredom and fatigue.

Your emotional functioning

Research has shown that people who exercise report that fitness has made them far more tolerant, relaxed and enthusiastic. It is interesting to note that many psychiatrists and psychologists now use exercise as an integral part of their treatment because they have found it can lift patients out of depression, often without the use of drugs.

Your quality of life

Active people have greater endurance and generally exude greater vitality. They find it a lot easier to change other lifestyle habits.

Your sex life

All the experts agree that working out will give your love life a real boost. Apart from all your new-found energy and muscle, exercise is thought to release hormones that give your libido a lift. Research has shown that the more people exercise, the more they want sex and the more they do it. Even once-a-week keep-fit warriors express improvements in their bed workouts.

The reasons for this are physical as well as psychological. Exercise puts you in touch with your body, you find you like the feel of your new body, and this will give you confidence. The body also releases endorphins during exercise which have a drug-like effect on some people. This results in a feeling of energy and euphoria, which may be directed into bed aerobics. As yet, there is no clinical evidence that endorphins stimulate the libido, but they do influence the levels of testosterone, the hormone which increases men's and women's sexual desires and particularly a woman's ability to reach orgasm. It is also said that women who have improved circulation are more easily aroused.

Don't get it wrong out there, starting a fitness regime isn't going to cure all the sicknesses known to man. You're still going to be prone to the occasional bout of bubonic plague, toothaches and the after-effects of being hit by a truck, but it's going to help with a lot of other problems in your temple.

Fitness makes you feel like you're master of your own lunacy.

Fatbusting Exercise

The exercises featured in this book are cardiovascular, circuit-training and body-strength exercises. All are geared to a whole-body approach with enough cardiovascular work to condition the heart and lungs and lose weight if so desired, enough strength work via hand-held weights and body weight to condition the muscles, and enough circuit-training to achieve ideal anaerobic conditioning (stamina). Throw in a pinch of flexibility work and enough variety to stop boredom, and what have you got, a class easy enough for anybody to do and hard enough to feel like you've had a serious workout.

The exercises fall into several categories.

Body-resistance training

The most readily available form of loading is the body itself. Using the body's weight allows you to do strength work during or after any other form of training, without any special equipment. A large range of different loads can be achieved by altering the resistance with a change of body position (like the different positions and leverage points of press-ups), or by the use of a partner.

Body resistance proves very effective for various types of strength work. However, consideration should be given to the type of exercise used, the effect required, the amount and nature of the resistance, the number of repetitions used and the quality of the movement.

Anaerobic exercise

Anaerobic exercise literally means without air. When applied to muscles this means 'without oxygen', and refers to the ways in which our muscles operate using other sources which they have in store. It is normally a supplement to the aerobic system, brought into action by the muscles during conditions with which the aerobic system can't cope alone. It shows up in three ways:

- At the beginning of a long exercise period, before the aerobic system has got fully into stride.
- In very explosive exercises.
- During intense bursts of activity.

Aerobic exercise

Aerobic literally means with air, and again the operative part of the air is oxygen. So aerobic endurance implies muscular work utilising oxygen to liberate the energy from the muscular fuels.

This is the most effective form of exercise for fat loss. For an exercise to be considered aerobic, it must involve large muscle group activity (not, contrary to popular belief, a large group activity!), it must be continuous (at least 15–20 minutes per session) and, for fat loss, it must fall within a certain heart-rate scale (see page 38).

Weight training

Muscular strength is generally built by encouraging the muscle or group of muscles concerned to exert a force while contracting

FAT FACT

Research suggests that exercise may be responsible for increasing the level of so-called good cholesterol (high-density lipoprotein). But, on the down note, exercise does not radically lower total serum cholesterol. A low-fat diet along with exercise is the best way to reduce cholesterol.

against a resistance (hand weights, dumbbells, sugar bags, benches etc). These contractions involve an increase in muscle tension. When this is repeated frequently, the muscles respond by accepting an increased flow of nutrients which in turn gives them the ability to deliver more power.

Circuit training

Circuit training combines aspects of weight training, strength work, aerobics and anaerobics, and is the Grandaddy of cross training.

Cross training

What is this? A new form of training designed to piss you off? A trendy new video designed to rake the money in or a form of training, sure to make you so cross that you give up exercising forever? Or is it the new poster, selling the new cross-training shoe, without which you can't exercise ever again?

Cross training has come into vogue during the 90s. Contrary to popular belief it wasn't an American concept, but has been around on the British fitness scene for years. Basically cross training is a combination of all you've encountered in the fitness world during the last decade, and that I've listed above. So what we have is a fitness regime that combines low- and high-impact movements, strength work using some form of resistance, circuit training, coordination skills and flexibility work. In other words, everything you wanted to know about sex but were too afraid to ask . . .

One of the major benefits of a cross-training class is that you're less likely to suffer stress-related injuries to the joints etc, due to the fact that you're not repeating constant movements on the same area of the body. Whether you attend low-impact, high-impact, circuit-training or weight-training classes, the sheer monotony of the movements causes structural damage, no matter how safe the class is.

Another point in favour of this form of training is that you can incorporate all the various aspects of fitness (flexibility, cardio-vascular work, skill and coordination, strength work and endurance) in the one class, as compared to limiting yourself to one or two of these in the average class.

Possibly the best aspect of this form of exercise is that you can cross over into other styles of exercise, for instance combining swimming with circuit training. As an example, swimming lengths of the pool, but every so often leaping out of the water and doing a small strength-based circuit to compensate for the fitness skills you miss just swimming. If you repeated this twice, gave it a fancy name like 'Surf and Turf', lo and behold, you would have a perfect example of cross training. So to hell with limiting yourself to one form of movement, and remember, 'Don't quit, just get cross'.

As Fatbusters is based entirely on cross-training theories, you can't go wrong. Apart from being real good for you, it's trendy and press-worthy. On a serious note, you can expect the following benefits from Fatbuster's workouts:

- An effective weight-loss programme, due to the concept of low-intensity exercise for weight loss (see page 40).
- A balance between aerobic and anaerobic training.
- A balanced strength development.
- A time-and-space efficient exercise programme.
- Routines that are easily adaptable for different ages and fitness levels.
- Routines that can be adapted for specific sport training if necessary.
- An effective fitness programme for rehabilitation if necessary.
- A low injury-risk exercise programme.
- A programme that's easy to do, and is more fun and demanding than the usual run-of-the-mill fitness class.

‘ Don't take up ballet if you move like a hippo; don't lambada if the only thing that swivels on your body is your dodgy knees. Gradual progression with each workout is expected, but don't run before you can walk, snakehips. ’

THE CASE STUDIES

I decided to stray from the usual with the case studies and actually give it to you as it is. No altered befores and afters, no subdued lighting and glam make-over jobs, no sucked-in stomachs, puffed-out chests and other magic tricks. For starters the four people I decided to use wouldn't be considered obese in purely cosmetic terms, but from health and fitness standards would be considered overweight (poor saps).

I generally find with most fitness-book case studies that they seem to use the biggest people they can get their hands on, have them lose outstanding amounts of weight in the shortest time possible, and then proclaim to the world that it's the only weight loss and fitness programme worth the paper it's written on. Don't take us for a bunch of idiots: the first ten stone is always easy, it's the last stone that separates the boys from the men. As for any author who claims they can lose twenty pounds of real weight in two weeks, they should change their job, climb the nearest mountain, grow a beard and wear a long flowing robe and work out how to divide five loaves of bread between the population of Central London.

So why does that make me any different? Well, for starters, the photos you see are the real thing, and the stories are from the case studies themselves, not the author's version of what he or she thought happened. And, lastly, what you see is what you get at the end of the day.

I picked the various people for the book for a number of reasons (the first being that they wanted their faces in a book). No, seriously, because I thought they represented a good cross-representation of society as I see it. For instance, Tracey from the waist up is in pretty good shape, but when it gets down to the lower half she is every woman's nightmare – solid thighs, bum and tum. Julian is what every Englishman abroad is like – Union Jack shorts and a massive belly (How big? Big enough to rest a pint on), long of leg and definitely thick in the head. As for the terrible two, Laura and Andrea: they're sisters of the same weight but totally different shapes – Laura 10 on the Richter Scale and Andrea managing a 6.5.

I set down a few rules for this term of 'Aerobics from Hell'.

● The posse had to think I was the best thing since sliced bread.

- They had to follow the exercise programme every day at home or attend a Fatbusters class. Slight deviations were allowed from the programme, depending on the posse's state of well-being in the morning (you know how it is after a night out on the booze).
- No-one was expected to diet at all during the programme, though gold stars where given to those who participated in good eating programmes (and hefty kicks up the backside for those who pigged out, Laura).
- Photographs were taken at the start of the programme and then twenty exercise sessions down the road.
- They were expected to give it their best throughout and the results prove they did. (These dudes could run the London Marathon at the drop of a hat and then still probably 'out-fit' me. It's a sorry state of affairs when your posse is fitter than you.)

Let's hand it over to the cast of this show and let them briefly explain their prior histories and what they felt about it at the end of the day, straight from the horses' mouth. The exciting thing with this programme is that life as you know it doesn't have to cease just because you want to lose some weight and get fit. The exercise loadings are so full that you can cover for the occasional blow-out now and again. Let's not get lost in all the mystique of fitness. Fitness is here so that you can enjoy your vices to the max. Take myself for instance: I smoke, eat pizza and drink beer and I'm not in bad shape. Fitness is great, it helps you enjoy life, not become your life. It's not the well of eternal youth, but you will be kicking until the last drink. Get on with it.

A last note. All the case studies have carried on with the programme since the initial stage, and I'm glad to report that Julian has traded his shorts in for a pair of lycras, and auditioned for the next Arnie movie. Tracey has just insured her pins for a million quid, Laura thinks she's a reincarnation of Bruce Lee, and Andrea has sent a letter to the London Monarchs saying next season she's going to kick butt and chew bubble gum and she's all out of bubble gum. No, seriously, they're all still at it – Fatbusters, the fast-acting, fat-burning exercise programme for fatties.

Tracey

I first got into fitness seriously about three years ago. I realised I had to do something about my weight and size when the elastic in my size 10–12 knickers was getting tight and cutting the blood off to my head. I wasn't really overweight, but I just felt uncomfortable with myself. So, I joined a West End gym. The only problem was you had to be made like a stick insect to become a member, and if you joined an aerobic class and broke out in a sweat you could get barred. . . . I knew then that I really needed to join a gym where size and shape didn't matter, somewhere you could be shown how to do a proper all-over body workout by someone who pushed you and didn't care how much you sweated. A friend told me about a gym just like that.

I went along one night and tried one of Jamie Addicoat's classes. Half-way through, I could hardly move my body from the horizontal

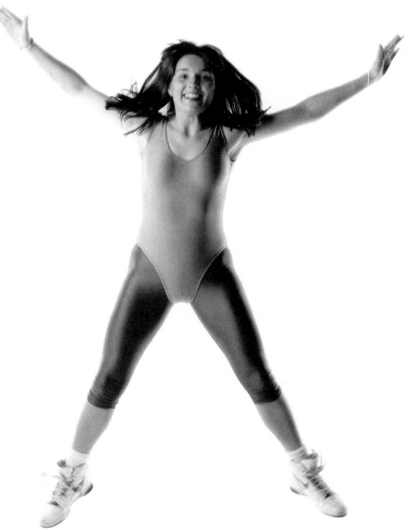

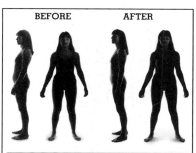

	BEFORE	AFTER
Waist	29 (INCHES)	26 (INCHES)
Hips	38	36
L. thigh	21½	20
R. thigh	21½	20
L. arm	11½	10½
R. arm	11½	11
Bust	35	34
Weight	132lbs (60.2kgs)	127lbs (57.9kgs)
Total inch loss		10½
Total weight loss		5lbs (2.3kgs)

position off the floor, and I thought it was an aqua aerobics class because of the sweat. I eventually got up because the teacher was shouting abuse at me. I then realised this was the one for me because this teacher really *could* put me through my paces.

Jamie screams, shouts and raves and works you to your max, and I've definitely noticed results over the last month. I've not lost much in weight (which is fine by me as there wasn't much to lose), but the inches

have come off and so my shape has changed (and, I might add, is still changing). I'm happy with this because I'm achieving what I started out to do.

I'm pleased I was asked to take part in the programme because I feel I've gained a lot from it. I don't think I would have carried on with it without Jamie's support and encouragement because, although I'm quite self-motivated when it comes to exercise, I still need that extra Addicoat push.

Julian

Thirty something, well, almost 29 years old, and getting ready to notch up another decade. Life has been good, I am happily married, two children and a successful career in retail. There was only one problem and that was my overall health and appearance. Over seven years of marriage I had forsaken taking regular exercise, and it showed. I was now carrying sixteen stone around with me. It wasn't that I hadn't exercised over the years, I had. You name it, I did it – body-building, American football, martial art and making babies. I would always start the same, find a club, pay the membership and then give it 100% effort for a couple of months before calling it a day. Something had to be done.

I had two choices: stay fat and unfit and not give a toss, or take the ultimate plunge and find the answer for me that would keep me on the thin and narrow. I picked up the telephone and spoke to Jamie, a colourful Aussie I had met earlier at a gym in Central London. He advised me about the infamous Fatbusters, a training regime of circuit, free weights, aerobics and his very own blend of verbal abuse.

I started. After a short time (a week to be precise), I began to feel the effects. The weight and inches started to do a runner and I was getting fit again. I trained full on five days a week at 7.30 am with the rest of the posse. I find the early-morning training sets me up for the rest of the day. Four weeks on, I feel great, leaner and meaner and still going strong. The one great thing about Addicoat's workouts is that anybody can do it, it's not poncey. I think I will survive more than two to three months on this one. The only problem is that when I get home in the evenings, I can hear the sound of my two daughters shouting '1, 2, 3'. They have now got in on the act doing exercises, members of Jamie's very own fan club. Is there no escape from this man?

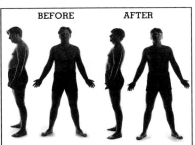

	BEFORE	AFTER
Waist	38 (INCHES)	33 (INCHES)
Hips	44	39
L. thigh	26	24½
R. thigh	25	23
L. arm	14½	13½
R. arm	15	13½
Chest	43	41
Weight	214lbs (97.6kgs)	200¼lbs (91.3kgs)
Total inch loss		18
Total weight loss		13¾lbs (6.3kgs)

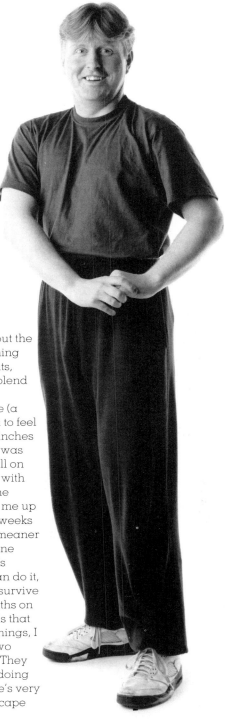

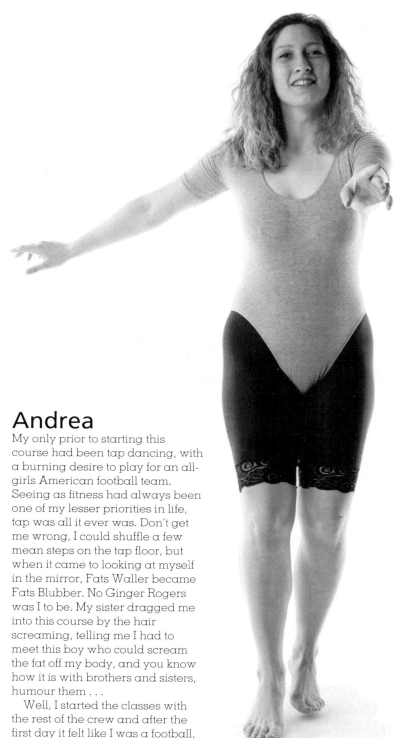

kicked all over the place just waiting for the final siren. I thought there's no way that I can do four weeks of this, this boy is a maniac. Laura kept me at it all week and it seemed to be getting a little better. It was like the fitness thing was taking off in great leaps and bounds, closely followed by some small noticeable body changes. It wasn't that stones were falling off, but my body was changing slightly, so I stuck it.

Well, four weeks down the road I still think that Jamie should be certified, but I'm a different lady, I've lost a few pounds, a load of inches and can run for a bus if need be. My tap has improved no end and Ginger Rogers I'm still not. But at least I'm not scared of the mirror anymore. I really enjoy this form of training to the point that I will stick with it for the next three score and ten, and I think I will try out for the London Monarchs next season. Thanks, Jamie, you're still a lunatic, but keep on doing what you do the best – frightening away fat forever.

Andrea

My only prior to starting this course had been tap dancing, with a burning desire to play for an all-girls American football team. Seeing as fitness had always been one of my lesser priorities in life, tap was all it ever was. Don't get me wrong, I could shuffle a few mean steps on the tap floor, but when it came to looking at myself in the mirror, Fats Waller became Fats Blubber. No Ginger Rogers was I to be. My sister dragged me into this course by the hair screaming, telling me I had to meet this boy who could scream the fat off my body, and you know how it is with brothers and sisters, humour them . . .

Well, I started the classes with the rest of the crew and after the first day it felt like I was a football,

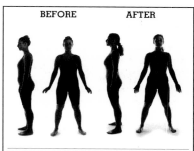

	BEFORE	AFTER
Waist	28 (INCHES)	26 (INCHES)
Hips	40	38
L. thigh	24	20
R. thigh	24	20
L. arm	10½	10½
R. arm	10	10
Bust	36	36
Weight	150lbs (68.4kgs)	141lbs (64.3kgs)
Total inch loss		12
Total weight loss		9lbs (4.1kgs)

Laura

I've never been able to stick to diets ever, basically because I'm a pig, and after about 5 minutes of low-cal, low-fat, low-taste and sparrow-sized portions, I want to fight the world. Armed with this feeling of irritability and the fact that cutting my food down didn't lose weight, I decided to try out Jamie's programme to see if it would make any difference.

I trained with my sister and Tracey in the morning so that I could leave the evenings free for karate (which I'm into fairly intensively). Motivation isn't a big thing with me, but training with the rest gave me that little bit extra. One of the major things about Fatbusters is that because it's a different workout every day, you can choose one to suit your mood on any given morning, great if you're feeling lazy. I've also got to add that even though I cut down on fats, I did have some major pig-outs, much to my disgust. Jamie was really cool about it as he kicked my behind.

So you can imagine my surprise when I actually started seeing changes in my body. The first was a dramatic improvement in my level of fitness, quickly followed by my strength which in turn improved my karate. But the biggest surprise was the inch loss. Even though I was ploughing through loads of food, good and bad, I was actually losing weight and inches. Not so much great amounts of pounds, but plenty on inches. I found this great for me. Just imagine eating and still bringing the inches down without the guilt. Every woman's wish come true. So I end this short note with thanks to Jamie Addicoat, fighter of obesity. I shall continue . . .

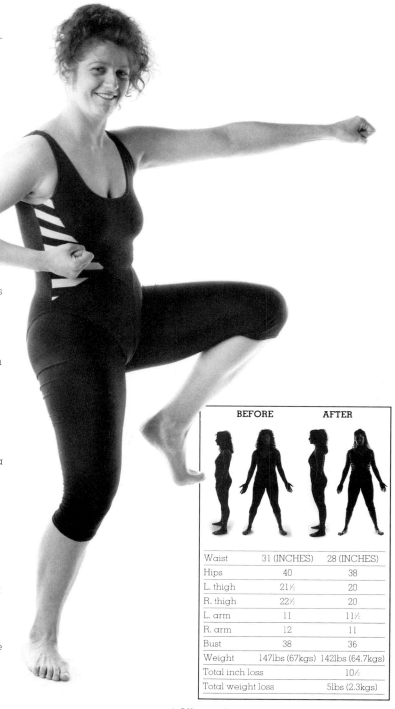

	BEFORE	AFTER
Waist	31 (INCHES)	28 (INCHES)
Hips	40	38
L. thigh	21½	20
R. thigh	22½	20
L. arm	11	11½
R. arm	12	11
Bust	38	36
Weight	147lbs (67kgs)	142lbs (64.7kgs)
Total inch loss		10½
Total weight loss		5lbs (2.3kgs)

* All weights are with clothing/shoes on

TESTING, TESTING AND MORE TESTING

A s the greatest cause of disease and death today is death and an abusive lifestyle, health evaluation and hazard appraisal tests rate your personal health habits, and guide you to make specific lifestyle changes to cut off disease before it starts. The underlying principle of these evaluations is the number of health hazards you face in life. Some are determined by age, sex, family history or ethnic background, while others are more closely associated with an individual's voluntary actions and habits. The answers you give to the questions and how you interpret the following tests, will forecast any major health risks you may have. The tests, though very basic, will give you an indication of your general physical evaluation. The first tests are for fun . . .

What Exercise Type Are You?

I get bored really easy

Generally your fitness worries are brought on very suddenly. It usually starts one morning when you realise you've lost one vital bodily function that you have taken for granted all your life, like the ability to tie your shoelaces from a standing position. It's not so much that you can't bend down and reach your feet, but more the fact that from a standing position you can't see your feet. You suddenly realise that your feet are totally obscured by your stomach. So instantly you panic and decide to do some fitness training.

Some of your character traits are:

- Worry a lot about whether you are fit or not.
- Know you are not fit and worry about it.
- Know you are not fit, don't worry about it, but know you should.
- Worry a lot about the economy, social issues and how to save the rainforest, but would really rather worry about being a couple of pounds overweight.

You're the exercise type who finds it all amazing at the beginning, but then finds it all a bit too much. You should try things like the London Marathon to start with as this only lasts for 8 hours at the most. Or you should try the latest fad exercise regime on video, as you can put this away on the shelf after one or two sessions. It seems that fitness appeals to you on the whole, but due to your small attention span, fitness soon loses its attraction. So if you fit this category, stick to exercise regimes that are interesting, in vogue, and stimulating. Learn loads of different forms of exercise regimes so that you can flit from one to the other at your leisure, never having to dwell on one form of exercise for more than 2 minutes at a time.

Lazy but means well

This character's fitness worries can be easily explained away by several reasons only understandable to themselves. On the whole, all the bodily functions of this person have reached the critical stage of no return. This doesn't seem to be a problem to this character type, because he/she thinks 'If I was meant to look like a Greek god, I would have been made out of marble, and anyway I have sufficient reasons not to become involved in too much exercise, even though I would love to'.

Some of this type's more common excuses might be:

- I will be better at resisting gamma and alpha ray penetration.
- I will be far more effective at sinking in quicksand, free-fall

parachute jumping and any other activities that require inter-action between body mass and gravity.

- I smile a great deal more than most people, as this is what's expected of me.

As you tend to mean well in attempting an exercise pro-gramme, try starting by walking to the front door at least three times per week, eventually stretching it out to 20 minutes per ses-sion, to make it aerobic. If this is still a bit too much for you, start with something slightly less active, like rising a few minutes earlier, and brushing your teeth more vigorously than usual. The calorie consumption of cleaning teeth is as follows:

- With a toothbrush and paste : 10 calories
- With toothbrush only : 26 calories
- With toothpaste only : 70 calories
- With a floor sander : 1000 calories

In all seriousness, start with the bare necessities of a fitness regime, and work up to brushing your teeth or other vigorous activities like breathing etc.

I've got no time

You have probably looked into the concept of getting fit at some stage in life and, like marriage, decided that fitness cannot be entered into wantonly or lightly. After contemplating all the pros and cons, you probably decided that, for better or worse, being a few stones overweight or being unable to run to the bus stop without taking two weeks' bedrest beforehand, was not as impor-tant as a rampant social or working life. You might even be in the 3% of the public, who can honestly confess that they have never worried about fitness during their life. The majority of people in this category, even though they haven't time to partake in an exercise regime, make amends in other ways:

- 60% start dieting.
- 15% give up smoking for 3 hours.
- 5% give up sex.
- 10% give up drinking for 3 hours.
- 5% take up smoking, sex and drinking.
- 2% take up something to get them arrested.

So, if you fit into this category, nothing I say will change your mind and divert you from your path of getting richer, having more children or becoming a bigger couch potato than you are already. You are probably an 'A'-type personality, forever on the move and very active in your day-to-day doings, as skinny as a praying mantis and need a fitness programme like a hole in the head. But have a thought for later on: we all slow down and gravity always wins in the end. So if you haven't got time now, think of later.

The disciplined person

What can be said about you that hasn't been documented already? You probably could liken yourself to the German race in your determination and whole-hearted pursuit of your fitness goals. You are so determined not to be swayed from your exercise programme, that things like showering, feeding the kids, kissing the spouse and feeding the dog really don't matter. Snow storms, tube strikes and even work will not stop you going for your evening run, or your class at 5am after the class at 10 the night before. Faced with the choice of your husband leaving, or you missing your gym workout, you don't even miss a beat as you help him pack his bags.

> **FAT FACT**
>
> 1 kg of body fat equals about 32,500 Kj (7600 Kcals) of energy. To use up this amount of energy you would have to run for 5 hours or jog for 11 hours.

Your disciplined approach to fitness has its drawbacks, like not being able to talk about anything apart from fitness, but you don't give a toss because you have the body of an 18-year-old, even though you're approaching 35. Your pancreas will probably survive 10 years after you've left this earth; if you were any tougher you would probably rust. Harder exercise regimes are your cup of tea, things that take commitment and skill, and loads of time.

What Body Type Are You?

On that note, it might be an idea to talk about the three body groups recognised by the establishment, as it's been discovered that certain training behaviour patterns identify with body types.

Genetics – the study of heredity and inherited characteristics – play a major part in the end result of your body shape. (Thank the EC for this standard requirement of all Europeans.) In layman's terms, if both your parents are gifted with short and stocky builds (broad hips and thick ankles), it's almost certain you're going to be gifted with at least some of these characteristics. Your body type will play a major role in your endeavours to change your body shape in the future.

Let's take a look at these body types, each of which has a distinct body shape and personality, and see if we can cross-relate them to your exercise type.

Ectomorph (hard gainer)

Ectomorphs are easily recognised by their long thorax and their short abdominal walls. In a fitness sense they are known for their stamina and endurance. You know the type, does three workouts and then some more; can, at the drop of a hat, run a mile and then pick up a squash racquet and play a 2-hour game without breaking into a sweat. I hate them.

Most ectos are small of frame, carry little body fat, and generally have a better overall shape than most dudes. It sounds like these bods don't need much doing to them, but they have one fairly large problem, their fitness rewards aren't on a par with the amount of work they need to do. As they are slow or hard gainers, their training will always be a long-term investment, and their body changes steady, rather than mind blowing. Due to their personality, they tend to be a little hyper, and need to slow down, possibly even changing their lifestyle down a gear or two. A few will get strung out waiting for quick results, but they must learn to relax and be patient, Rome wasn't built in a day. Programme-wise, they should stick to short, fast intense workouts with a demanding workload for the best results.

Mesomorph (easy achiever)

God's chosen ones, a bit like the Twelve Tribes of Israel. This body was possibly in good shape from early days, and is probably a dab hand at most things it attempts. This is the kind of person who makes half-hearted attempts at exercise, but lo and behold the muscles grow and weight drops off before your eyes. (The kind of person you love to hate.) They could probably lose weight on a 14-pint-a-day-and-vindaloo-curry diet. Exercise-wise, they are fairly laid back about their exercise, and often do whatever the mood takes them. The only fault they have is that they do not exploit their full potential.

FAT FACT

———— ● ————

To ward off the effects of gravity, you've got to keep good breast muscle tone. Exercise is definitely the answer, but from a food point of view eat loads of low-fat proteins, the nutrient which builds and maintains strong firm muscles.

———— ● ————

Endomorph (very easy gainer)

Endomorphs are the opposite to Ectomorphs, in that they gain weight easily, and have the tendency to be constantly overweight. Endomorphs belong to the group who have inherited large bones and big frames. They lack motivation, and need constant encouragement. By nature, they are usually easy-going. Training wise, they require a high amount.

Which one are you? See if you can match your exercise type to your body type, and work out your kind of exercise person.

Okay, so you answered your questions, now it's time to move on to the actual tests. Proceed with care as some of you might find the testing a workout in itself. Compile all your results and find out where you are lacking. When and if you start Fatbusting, put that little bit more effort into the areas you are lacking in, and watch the change over the period of the course. At the end of your six weeks, try the fitness testing again, and see for yourself why Fatbusting is here to stay!

A point to remember about pre-test requirements. Do not eat or drink caffeinated drinks in the 2 hours proceeding your actual tests, as you will effect some of the results. Also bear in mind that some of yesterday's exercise efforts (if any), or even yesterday's workload, might affect today's results. An adequate warm-up and cool-down should be used preceding and following the tests: for example, flexibility testing should be preceded by stretching (see page 69) to avoid injury to the muscles and joints.

A last thought to bear in mind before progressing any further is that the fitness testings in this book are only a general guideline. Most tests available today, even the best, can be subject to a 5% deviation either side. Try not to make decisions that may affect your results. Remember you are not a doctor or God. Giving yourself a complete go-ahead based on your results can be lethal. Proceed slowly and surely, because acquiring health and fitness is a gradual progressive process, at all levels, from the beginner to the advanced participant. If you have any doubts whatsoever, see your doctor or your local fitness trainer.

All right, troops, get cracking with the tests, and see if you're man or woman enough to Fatbust.

The Ten Steps to Self Assessment

1. Answer the health evaluation and hazard appraisal questions – in the Medical and Exercise Profiles – to determine if you should consult your doctor before beginning the fitness tests and starting the fitness programme.

2. If you do not fall into any of the risk categories, you can proceed with the tests. If you can demonstrate any of the risks listed, you should be medically evaluated and receive consent from your doctor before proceeding.

3. Once cleared, it's your last chance to decide if you're going to proceed. It's a bit like Monopoly: if you don't go past Go, you don't receive 200 press-ups.

4. Take the Passive Fitness Tests, temperature, pulse and blood pressure. Make sure your temperature is fine, check your pulse to determine your training heart-rate zone (very important, this), and have your blood pressure taken.

5. If all three Passive Fitness Tests are normal, proceed to the fitness testing. If you have a high temperature, postpone until you feel normal. If you show signs of high blood pressure and have not received medical clearance to exercise, forget it.

6. Carry out the Submaximal Test.

7. Carry out the Flexibility Measurement Tests.

8. Carry out the Muscle Endurance Tests.

9. Do the Body Fat Measurement Tests.

10. Assess the results and determine the major areas that you need to work on.

Best of luck, dudes!

Medical Profile

Answer these questions honestly. If 'yes' is the answer to one or more, seek your doctor's advice as to whether you should commence an exercise regime.

- Have you ever had any diagnosed orthopaedic conditions, injury, illness, back or joint problem that may be aggravated by exercise?
- Have you ever had arthritis, asthma, diabetes, epilepsy, hernia, dizziness, gout, circulation or stomach conditions?

- Have you ever had high or low blood pressure, rheumatic fever, a stroke or high cholesterol levels?
- Have you ever had any diagnosed cardiac condition, or any direct family history of it, heart palpitations or murmurs, or general pains in the chest?
- Are you now pregnant, or have you recently been pregnant?
- Have you ever had any serious medical condition or surgery?
- Have you ever had any serious lung condition?
- Do you smoke or work with heavy smokers? Have you ever smoked? How long did you smoke for?
- Are you at present on any form of medication, or taking any form of recreational drugs?
- Is there any factor at all that might be reason to prevent the commencement of an exercise regime (apart from the fact you don't want to do it)?

Exercise profile

If possible, consult with a qualified fitness person when answering your exercise-related questions, and, more importantly, when compiling your fitness testing results in the next few pages.

- Were you involved in exercise or sport at school?
- Are you at present involved in any form of sport or regular exercise? (For exercise to be considered regular, you must do at least three sessions a week for an absolute beginner, graduating to five sessions.)
- How would you describe your present physical condition?
  Sickly • Fat • Unfit • Healthy • Fit • Animal •
- What are the main benefits you want from an exercise programme?
  Fat loss • Muscular tone • Fitness • Maintaining a level of fitness • Good health • Sport specific • Or just for the crack •

There are no real 'yes' or 'no' interpretations here, just common sense. If you do start an exercise regime after your fitness tests, do so at a sensible pace, as you are responsible for your own well-being. Remember, it's taken years to get into the shape you are now, it ain't going to disappear overnight, and you're not sixteen years old any more.

Taking Your Temperature

Using a clinical thermometer, shake the mercury towards the bulb at the end with a few downward flicks of the wrist. Make sure the mercury level is below the point indicating the normal temperature of 37°C (98.6°F). Put the bulb under the tongue, close the lips (not the teeth!), and leave for 1–2 minutes. You can be 0.5°C (1°F) above or below the normal temperature, but anything higher, and you could be unwell. Do not continue with the tests.

Resting Heart Rate and Taking Your Pulse

In the following few paragraphs lies the whole theory of Fatbusters, so read carefully!

A great variation occurs in the resting heart rate in any one person, at any given one time. It's like a yo-yo. Most people have a resting heart rate of between 70 and 90 beats per minute, although it can be elevated by such things as smoking, stress, temperature, humidity, digestion, spicy foods (so watch the curries) and medications, to name but a few. A high resting heart rate can also be a sign of a poor state of fitness.

FAT FACT

●

Very few people have a low metabolic rate. According to the latest studies, fatter people generally have a higher metabolic rate than the skinnies.

●

Resting heart rate can be measured by several methods, but we will use the plain old method of taking your pulse. The pulse can be found at several body locations where arteries are close to the skin's surface. The one we will use is the inside of the wrist in line with your thumb. This radial pulse corresponds directly to the contraction and relaxation of the left ventricle of the heart, so provides the most accurate reading.

- Find your pulse with your index and middle fingers placed on the thumb side of the wrist. (Never use the thumb to find your pulse, as it has a slight pulse of its own.)
- Count the number of beats in 1 minute (or the number of beats in 10 seconds and multiply by six). This gives you your resting heart rate in beats per minute.

By the way, after you begin an aerobic-based exercise programme, it is common to see a *decrease* in your resting heart rate. The reasons (for the technical buffs), are an increased stroke volume, enhanced delivery of oxygen to the muscles and increased oxidative capabilities on the cellular level, allowing

YMCA NORMS FOR RESTING HEART RATE

	Percentile	Resting heart rates (applicable to adults of all ages)	
		Male	Female
Excellent:	95%	52	59
	85%	59	63
	75%	65	68
Average:	50%	72	73
	30%	78	80
	15%	84	85
Poor:	5%	93	92

(Adapted from *Y's Way to Fitness*, The YMCA of USA, Chicago, 1982)

for efficient oxygen utilisation. In other words, the more you exercise your heart and lungs, the more conditioned they become, and the heart has to work less hard to do its work.

For almost everyone, any exercise, especially aerobic exercise (there's that word again), makes your heart speed up from its normal resting rate. (Think of how it thumps when you run for the bus.) But too much exercise, or too intense a level of exercise, can be bad, making your heart beat far too fast, so you need to find your own training level which should be neither too comfortable nor too strenuous.

To find this training level you need, I'm afraid, to be a bit of a mathematician. Subtract your age from 220 for the predicted maximum heart rate. Then, most importantly, calculate the number that is 65% of that. If you're 35 years old, for instance, it's 220 minus 35 = 185; 65% of 185 = 120. Therefore, 120 heart or pulse beats per minute is that person's training level – to start with.

It's only when you *first* enter a fitness programme that your target heart rate should be at 65% of the predicted maximum heart rate. Eventually, after progression and time, your target heart rate – because of your increasing fitness – can be increased to 75%, and then 85% if it can be tolerated. Please note, however, that for the cardiac rehab person, those with severe hypertension, or individuals who are extremely unfit or overweight, a starting figure of 50% of the maximum heart rate would be more desirable.

The following scale may be of help to you to find your target heart rate.

PREDICTED TARGET HEART RATES				
AGE	MAX. H.R.	*x* 65%	*x* 75%	*x* 85%
20–29	200–191	130–124	150–143	170–162
30–39	190–181	123–118	142–135	161–154
40–49	180–171	117–111	135–128	153–145
50–59	170–161	110–104	127–120	144–137

Think back to aerobic exercise. Remember I said that fat was used as a primary fuel source during such exercising? Well, research has shown that a greater proportion of fat is used as fuel for the exercise if the intensity of the exercise is *low* – and this is where Fatbusters comes in.

Exercise which produces a heart rate of 65–85% of the predicted maximum heart rate is Fatbusting, particularly at the lower end of the range. I know you can't have your fingers on your pulse all the time – although at the beginning it's useful in self-assessment – but there's also an easier method. If you become breathless during the exercise, this would indicate that the aerobic threshold has been reached, and that the exercise is probably too intense for effective fat loss. The exercise should be continued at a 'conversational pace', ie you should be able to talk at any time during your exercise programme.

All this will come up again and again, so commit it very thoroughly to memory!

> **FAT FACT**
>
> Keep the stomach flat by eating little amounts throughout the day, instead of two or three massive meals. Stomachs are stretched by vast quantities of food. Keep to low-fat diets for the best-looking stomach around, and exercise won't go astray. Bloated stomachs can result from water retention, so cut down on salt in the diet. Vitamin C is great for combating water retention.

Have Your Blood Pressure Taken

You will need to consult your doctor to obtain your blood-pressure readings, but a brief outline of what it is may be helpful.

Blood pressure is the lateral pressure exerted against the walls of a blood vessel. It is measured in units (mm Hg) at various times throughout the cardiac cycle due to the changing pressures at different points in the cycle. The highest pressure is referred to as the systolic pressure, the lowest pressure as the diastolic pressure. The difference between the two numbers is referred to as the pulse pressure. A typical blood pressure is 120/80 mm Hg.

The exact figures used to describe hypertension – or high

blood pressure – vary considerably, depending on the source, but most people tend to agree on 145/95 mm Hg or higher as being borderline high blood pressure. This normally requires medical treatments which lessen the demands on the heart, reducing cardiac output (usually beta blockers). A far healthier approach is to reduce body weight and body fat. This should be done via a combination of exercise and diet. (It's probably a good idea to reduce salt intake too.)

Be sure the doctor knows *why* you are having your blood pressure taken, and that he passes you as fit, because high blood pressure and exercise do not go together.

Submaximal Test

One of the major benefits of exercise is increased heart and lung endurance, which allows you to do more for a longer period of time at a faster pace. As exercises to improve the working capacity of the heart and lungs are part of most fitness regimes, an aerobic testing is an important aspect of your fitness assessment.

At present there are two forms of testing for cardiovascular or cardio-respiratory fitness. Maximal exercise testing measures maximal aerobic capacity, and requires total effort to the point of voluntary exhaustion. This form of testing is extremely accurate, but requires a high level of motivation on your behalf and should be conducted under controlled conditions with trained fitness consultants.

The testing that is more suitable for you at home is submaximal testing. Submaximal tests require you to perform at approximately 65–85% of heart rate reserve for a set time, and to finish before exhaustion. Your heart rate is taken either during or immediately after the test. The percentiles are based on the assumptions that a relationship exists between heart rates, oxygen consumption and workloads. Submaximal testings are not as accurate as maximal testings, but are much easier and much safer to perform.

The submaximal test that we are going to use is the 3-minute

FAT FACT

●

TRUE OR FALSE:

1. Jogging for 2 miles has a greater calorie expenditure than walking the same distance at a brisk lively pace?
● FALSE: Mile for mile, walking briskly has the same calorie burn as jogging. You just get there faster jogging.

2. 2 oz crinkle-cut chips has the same calorific count as the same amount of thick-cut chips?
● FALSE: Crinklies weigh in at about 80 calories per 2 oz, while thick-cut chips weigh in at 40 calories per 2 oz.

3. In expenditure of energy, lean muscle tissue burns more calories than fat?
● TRUE: Each pound of lean muscle tissue requires about an extra 50–100 calories per day to be a good boy.

●

step test (devised by Dr Fred Kasch). All you will need is a 12 inch (30 cm) bench or step, and a watch. All you are required to do is step up and down on to the bench at approximately 24 steps per minute for 3 minutes. The sequence should be right foot up, then left, right foot down and then left and carry on. When stepping on to the bench make sure the feet are flat on the bench.

If at any stage during the test you feel dizzy, faint, nauseous, short of breath, or you just need to stop . . . stop.

Once you complete the 3-minute test, sit yourself down and proceed to take your pulse (see page 38) for 1 minute. This post-exercise heart rate reflects your cardiovascular ability to recover from exercise. Then compare this to the table below which lists the norms established for men and women aged 20 to 46.

FAT FACT

An apple has 101 calories, and you would need to jog for approximately 10 minutes to work it off. A piece of cake has around 400 calories, and you would have to jog for nearly 40 minutes to work them off.

1-MINUTE RECOVERY HEART RATES		
	Men	**Women**
	(20–46)	(20–46)
Excellent	81–90	79–84
Good	99–102	90–97
Above average	103–112	106–109
Average	120–121	118–119
Below average	123–125	122–124
Fair	127–130	129–134
Poor	136–138	137–145

(Adapted from *Y's Way to Fitness*, The YMCA of USA, Chicago, 1982)

There may be as much as 10–20% error in estimating VO2 Max (your maximal aerobic capacity) using the step test. Also under any workload, oxygen uptake can vary as much as 15% between various people. However, this test is still a very good indicator of cardio-respiratory endurance. As you get fitter, as your heart and lungs become more conditioned, you will recover from an exercise session quicker, so it stands to reason that follow-up tests will show a lower recovery heart rate.

Flexibility Measurement Tests

Flexibility is the range of motion possible at all joint areas of the body. In practical terms, it means the ability to move. No person is exempt from lack of flexibility, tightness and tension, including those who throw their legs all over the place at the ballet, but I guess putting your head between your legs could come in handy at some stage in life.

No, on a serious note, as flexibility allows us to move comfortably and more easily, it must be one of the more important fitness goals, contrary to popular belief. Without a degree of flexibility, working out will be that much harder.

There are four basic flexibility tests. Mark down your results to evaluate later.

Front reach

Front reach flexibility tests the range of motion through the lower back and the back of the legs (hamstrings).

- Sit on the floor with your legs straight out in front of you and feet flat against the side of a small box. Tape a ruler to the top of the box with the 6 inch (15 cm) mark lined up at the edge of the box.
- Reach forward along the ruler.
- Record the spot on the ruler where your middle finger reaches.
- The 6 inch (15 cm) mark on the ruler lined up with the box's edge is the 'O' mark. If you reach 2 inches (5 cm) short of the 'O' mark, you score a minus 2. If you stretch 2 inches (5 cm) past the mark, score yourself a plus 2.

Rate yourself according to the following scale.

FRONT REACH SCALE	
Inches (cm)	**Rating**
−5 (−13) or less	very poor
−4 to −1 (−10 to −2.5)	poor
0	fair (touching toes)
+1 to +3 (+2.5 to +7.5)	moderate
+4 to +6 (+10 to +15)	good
+7 to more (+18)	excellent

Back arch

The back arch test measures flexibility throughout the back. You will need someone to help you measure.

- First you must sit flat on the floor keeping the back straight and the feet out in front. Measure the distance from the chin to the floor. This is the sitting height and should be recorded.
- Lie face down on the floor with legs crossed over at the ankles and hands clasped on the small of the back. Using your lower back muscles, stomach and buttocks, lift your upper body off the ground but make sure you keep your hips down.
- Measure the distance from the centre of the collarbone to the floor and note this down.
- Now divide the back arch figure by the sitting height to come up with a percentage score.

Rate yourself according to the following scale.

BACK ARCH SCALE	
Percent	**Rating**
10% or less	Very poor
20%	Poor
30%	Fair
40%	Moderate
50%	Good
60% or more	Excellent

Leg stretch

This test is a quick and easy measurement of the flexibility of the back of the body including the backs of the legs (hamstrings).

- Stand flat-footed with the feet slightly apart for balance.
- With knees slightly bent, roll the upper part of the body down and try to touch the floor with the fingers (or the palms if you can manage). Then straighten the legs. No bouncing on the stretch. Let gravity do the work.

Rate yourself according to the following scale.

LEG STRETCH SCALE	
Stretch	**Rating**
Fingers don't touch floor	Poor
Fingers touch floor	Good
Palms rest flat on floor	Excellent

Upper torso

This measures the flexibility of the waist upwards.

- Tape an 'X' on the wall at about shoulder height.
- Stand with your back centred to the 'X', about a foot from the wall.
- Twist the upper body to the left (do not move the feet) and touch the 'X' with both hands, then reverse and twist to the right and do the same to be sure the mark is reachable.
- Start counting the number of times you hit the 'X' with both hands, alternating from left to right, in 30 seconds.

Rate yourself according to the following scale.

UPPER TORSO SCALE	
Hits	**Rating**
0–5	Poor
6–12	Good
13–17	Excellent

Remember, never force any of your stretches with a ballistic (bouncing) motion. Be gentle. Stretching should be easy, not painful.

Muscle Endurance Tests

Muscular endurance is about how much strength the muscle can produce at any given moment. It is measured by how powerful a contraction a particular muscle or muscle group can produce on demand. The test is important, so that you can discover your areas of need and apply specific exercises to develop strength in these areas.

Press-ups

The press-up determines upper body endurance.

- Kneel down on the floor on all fours. Make sure the hands are shoulder width apart, facing forward. Keeping your back straight, bend from the hips lowering your nose to the floor. Never lock out the elbows, and then return to the starting position. Always pay particular attention to keeping the hands in line with the shoulders at all times. Never sag the lower back or arch the upper back.

● Perform as many press-ups as possible. There is no time limit. You stop when you can't possibly do another press-up.

Rate yourself according to the following scale.

PRESS-UP SCALE	
Press-ups	**Rating**
0 – 5	Poor
6 – 10	Fair
11–15	Average
16–30	Good
31 or more	Excellent

Sit-ups

The sit-up tests the endurance of the abdominal muscles.

● Lie on the floor on your back with your hands on the side of your head. Don't pull on the neck. The knees should be bent with the feet flat on the floor.

● Pull yourself up as far as you can, using your abdominals, to the point of maximum muscle contraction. Keep the lower back on the floor at all times.

● Uncurl back to the resting position.

● Continue until fatigue prevents you from doing any more.
  Rate yourself according to the following scale.

SIT-UP SCALE	
Sit-ups	**Rating**
0 – 5	Poor
6 – 9	Fair
10–20	Average
21–35	Good
36 and over	Excellent

Knee-bends

The knee-bend tests the endurance of the leg muscles.

● Stand erect, and bend your knees to lower the body to the ground, using the muscles of the upper legs. The back must remain straight.

● Stop your descent at the point just before the heels leave the ground, then start to push back up again.

● Carry on until you cannot return to the starting position after the knee-bend.

Rate yourself according to the following scale.

KNEE-BEND SCALE	
Knee-bends	Rating
0 – 15	Poor
16 – 25	Fair
26 – 30	Average
31 – 36	Good
36 onwards	Excellent

Body Fat Measurement Tests

As body weight is not a clear indicator of fatness, you need to determine the ration of lean muscle tissue to body fat. As you won't have the equipment generally used on body composition tests these days, we will use 'the pinch test'. Bear in mind this style of testing is not as accurate as the new styles of testings available today, but it will give you a fair estimate of your body-fat percentage.

Before going any further with the test, it might be an apt time to explain the differences between overfat, overweight and obesity or fat, fat and fatter.

Overfat

Overfat basically means having excessives stores of body fat.

Overweight

Overweight basically means you weigh more than the normal standards given by height to weight charts. This doesn't necessarily mean that you are overweight, because these charts tend to be misleading, due to the fact that they measure pounds of body weight not body fat.

For example, heavily muscled athletes would be considered overweight according to standard charts, when in actual fact they are generally far leaner because they have minimal body fat. On the other hand, I've dealt with fashion models who are considered very skinny, but who have large percentages of body fat, far larger in fact than the average so-called fat person, because they have lost the wrong kind of weight.

Obese

Obese is what every woman in the world thinks she is. No, seriously, obesity is the technical term to describe your degree of overfat. Most research says that obesity is being more than 5% fatter than the average dude of your age and sex. So if the average proportion of body fat for young men is 15% and young woman 25%, and you are either 25% or more (young men) or 30% or more (young women), you are what's considered a fattie.

BODY-FAT PERCENTAGE LEVELS		
Classification	Men	Women
What's needed to exist	5%	8%
Fat levels for good performance	5–13%	12–22%
Fat levels for health	10–25%	18–30%
Overfat	More than 25%	More than 30%

So, let's march on and see if we make the fatties of the world.

The pinch test

- Have a friend do the pinching and measuring (make sure it's a friend, because we don't want any laughing at this stage), as you probably won't be able to measure your skinfold yourself.
- Let the right arm hang down at your side. The skinfold site is on the back of the upper arm midway between the shoulder and the elbow.
- Pull a vertical fold of skin between the thumb and first finger. Pull away the skin and fat, not any muscle (that's the hard stuff).
- Measure with a ruler the thickness of the fold to the nearest ¼ inch (5 mm), between the thumb and forefinger. Sometimes the outer portion of the skinfold is thicker than the flesh between the fingers. To avoid this, make sure the fold is level with the side of the thumb. Do not press the ruler against the skinfold, as this will flatten it out and make it thicker than it is.
- Take two measurements, releasing the skinfold between each measurement, and record the average of the two measurements.
- Estimate percentage of body fat from the chart opposite.

FAT FACT

With the boom in fitness and good eating, you would think that the average Brit would be getting slimmer and fitter. Wrong. The latest research shows that the average person is a fat and unfit slob, and that women's dress sizes have moved up two notches from size 12 to size 14.

ESTIMATED PERCENTAGE OF BODY FAT		
	Fat percentage	
Skinfold thickness	Men	Women
¼ inch (5 mm)	5–9%	8–13%
½ inch (1.25 cm)	9–13%	13–18%
¾ inch (1.75 cm)	13–18%	18–23%
1 inch (2.5 cm)	18–22%	23–28%
1½ inch (3.75 cm)	22–27%	28–33%
2 inches (5 cm)	27–32%	33–38%
2½ inches (6.25 cm)	32–37%	38–43%

Generally fat comprises more than a quarter of the total body weight of most people. The ideal amount of body fat for an active healthy male is 12% and the average healthy, active female with slender figure should be striving for 18% body fat.

Now you have found out a lot about yourself, medically and physically. Assess the results and determine the major areas on which you need to work. The Fatbusting course covers six weeks, divided into 30 days of work and 12 days of rest (that is, you repeat each week six times). This should help you lose up to 14 lb (6 kg) – or more. I can only wish you luck!

‘ *The single largest concern for all the fatties of the world is how to change their body shape in the least possible time, and with the least possible effort. In most cases, the good news is that it can happen. The bad news is that it won't happen overnight, and it will take loads of blood, sweat and tears.* ’

THE WARM-UP AND COOL-DOWN

Before an exercise workout, you must undergo a warm-up; after the workout, you must undergo a cool-down. Both of these are vital for safety, but first we must consider posture. Sloppy habits, shyness and poor muscle tone all eat away at our ability to stand, sit and walk well. Can you carry it off, wearing that new cut-away bikini, or have you developed a back that the hunchback of Notre Dame would be proud of? Posture is really important as it can contribute quite significantly to your ability to perform exercise correctly.

Sorting your posture out might as well begin indulgently – with a massage. A massage restores circulation to cramped-up areas, and coaxes muscles into longer, more relaxed darlings. A massage or two reminds you of what it feels like to be an upstanding citizen again.

Then the next step is to train yourself to sit properly once more. You know, back straight, feet flat on the floor, knees at an 90° angle etc.

The step following that is to exercise the back and stomach muscles which in due course will improve the tone of these areas.

Posture

Back Raises

Lie face down on the floor with forearms resting on the floor in front of you. Raise your chest slightly from the floor, and then raise first one leg, then the other. Feel the muscles of the lower back tighten slightly. Do not hyper-extend the lower back. It's only necessary to raise the chest and legs a few inches off the ground.

Reps: 10 for everyone.

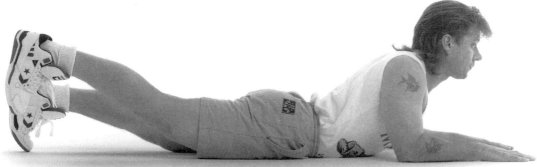

Posterior Flys

Lie face down on the floor, with hands stretched out at right angles to the body. Keeping chest and feet on the ground, lift hands and arms. Don't let your hands move back, maintain the 90° angle of arms to body.

Reps: 25 for everyone.

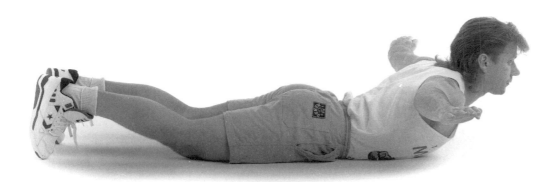

POSTURE

Lat Rows

Stand with knees slightly bent, and lean forward from the hips so that the upper body is at a 90° angle to your legs. Hold a light weight or a can of soup in your left hand, and lift the weight from your right hand to your left underarm.
Reps: 25 on each side.

Stomach Crunches

Lie on your back with knees bent and arms by the side of your head. Lift knees and cross ankles. With chin tucked in, gently lift the shoulder blades off the ground, hold for 1 second and lower back without letting your upper torso touch the ground.
Reps: 20 for everyone.

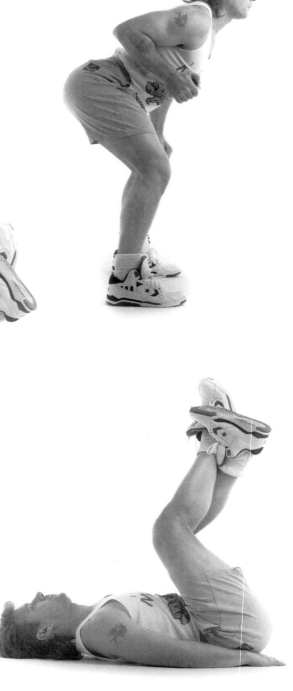

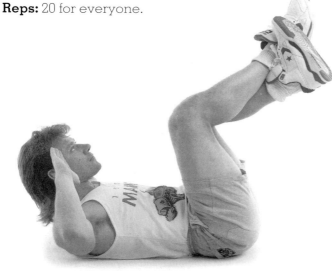

Reverse Stomach Crunches

Lie on your back with the knees tucked into your chest, ankles crossed, and hands lying beside your body. Use your hands and stomach to lift your hips off the ground, hold for 1 second and lower. Don't roll your hips towards your head, but lift them upwards.
Reps: 20 for everyone.

POSTURE

Many British health writers describe the exercise which is deemed most specific to improving your posture and for feeling what good posture is. With hands on hips, stand with your heels 2 inches (5 cm) away from the wall, with your head, shoulders, elbows and buttocks against the wall. Pull in your stomach and tighten your buttocks, while gently rotating your pelvis forwards until the curve of your lower back flattens against the wall (you'll have to bend your knees slightly). Tilt slowly backwards and forwards ten times, then, holding the position, slide down the wall a foot or two, and gently come back up again, trying to keep all those parts still pressed against the wall. Do this exercise twice daily.

And, before you proceed with any warm-up or workout, particular attention should be paid to posture and positioning of yourself during specific exercises, particularly leg and stomach exercises, as these are the ones that can be performed totally wrongly. They can cause permanent damage if performed incorrectly for any great length of time.

Posture for Leg Exercises and Weight-training

When performing leg exercises, always stand with feet shoulder-width apart, and with knees soft (with a slight bend). The knees should always point over the feet. The only variation on this would be feet together, but again the knees would be soft and in line with the feet.

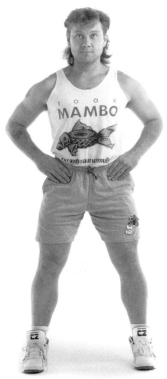

The pelvis is tilted slightly forward, the stomach held tight, and the chest lifted high. The head and back should be in one straight line, and bent slightly forward.

Breathing has always been a point of contention with everyone, but I think you should just breathe naturally. Do *not* stop breathing, as you tend to die.

POSTURE

Posture for Abdominal Work

The basic position for all abdominal work is lying on your back, consciously pushing your spine into the floor, so the lower back stays flat throughout all of the movement. The knees are bent up, feet flat on the floor and hip distance apart.

If lifting the head up, either frame the face with your hands, pressing the elbows back, or touch the sides of your head with your fingertips, again pressing the elbows back, or support the back of your head with your hands, once more pressing your elbows back. When you lift, the head, upper back and shoulders should come off the ground, but the lower back is still pressed into the floor.

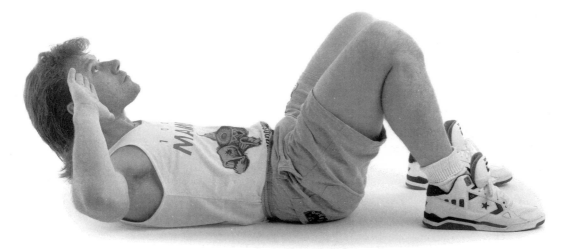

The Warm-Up

The aim of the warm-up is:

- To prepare the joints of the body for exercise.
- To prepare the heart and lungs for exercise, by increasing the muscle core temperature and blood flow to the muscles.
- To prevent the chances of muscle soreness and injury.
- To prepare the body's neuromuscular response patterns.

To achieve all this, we include:

- Exercises that provide for the release of tension and stress.
- Exercises that gradually increase in intensity.
- Exercises that utilise all body segments and all the major muscle groups.
- Exercises that raise the heart rate rapidly.

You should always avoid any time-lag between the warm-up and the workout, and workout and cool-down. And you must always leave time for your warm-up, even though you are pushed.

The body is affected in various ways during the warm-up:

- Body temperature increases gradually.
- The rate of exchange between oxygen in the blood and cells increases.
- The warm-up gives the body time to transport extra blood from areas that don't need it as much, to the areas that will need it later in the workout.
- The heart, metabolic and respiratory rates are raised, so that, as demands are made on these systems, no discomfort should be felt.
- Synovial fluid becomes more rapidly available to the joints, ligaments, tendons and connective tissues, making them more flexible. Therefore increasing the range of motion, hence protecting the body against injury.
- The deep muscle temperature increases, which in turn decreases internal friction within the muscles. Due to increased temperature inside the muscles, the muscles can contract and relax with greater speed, which in turn leaves the muscles prepared for harder workloads without risk of injury.
- If during the warm-up, exercises that are related to the main workouts are mimicked, the body will rehearse and facilitate the following workout's neuromuscular response patterns.
- The warm-up will prepare you physiologically for what you are about to receive.

WARM-UP

Now it's time to move on to the warm-up and flexibility section of your workouts. The warm-up should be performed before any of the workouts in this book. Use the same warm-up for all the workouts, and any other forms of exercise you might consider doing. Allow 10–12 minutes per workout for the warm-up. This time span might decrease slightly as you get fitter. If you find it too easy in time, increase the number of reps per exercise or bump up the intensity slightly, but remember it's only the warm-up and not the workouts.

Note: Always keep movements fluid, don't bounce or jerk. Use music to help motivate you. Exclude use of arms if you find it difficult to coordinate arms and legs.

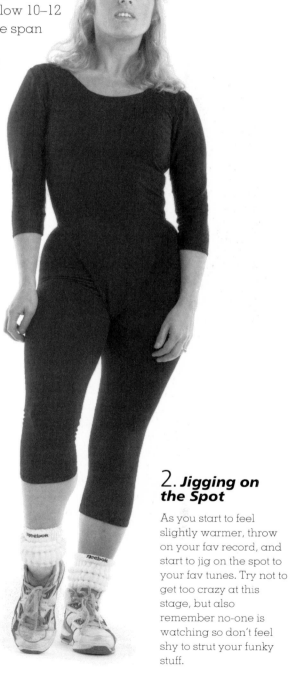

1. *Walking around the Room*

These first few exercises are the First Pulse Raiser, designed to raise the pulse slightly. Start walking around the room. Increase the length of your stride and pump your arms into the air and to the front and sides at your leisure. Occasionally pump your arms more vigorously to elevate your pulse. Every so often walk in the opposite direction to counteract the forward stress.

2. *Jigging on the Spot*

As you start to feel slightly warmer, throw on your fav record, and start to jig on the spot to your fav tunes. Try not to get too crazy at this stage, but also remember no-one is watching so don't feel shy to strut your funky stuff.

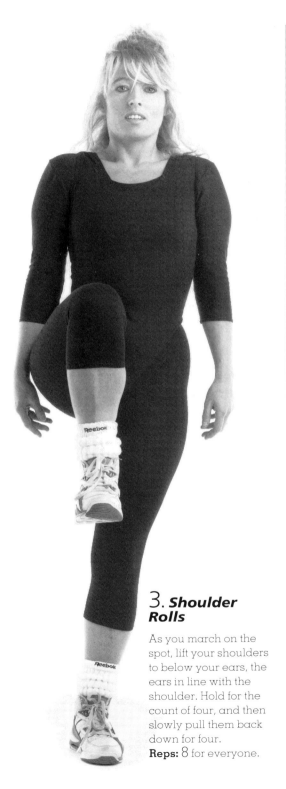

4. Head Tilts and Chin Forward

Starting Position: Stand, feet shoulder width apart, knees soft, hands on hips (A).
Movement: Tilt your left ear towards your left shoulder (B), then return to the starting position before pressing your right ear towards your right shoulder.
Reps: 8 times to each side.
After finishing the head tilts, push your chin towards your chest, and then back to starting position. Under no circumstances bend your neck backwards.
Reps: 8 for everyone.

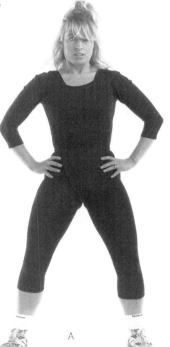

A

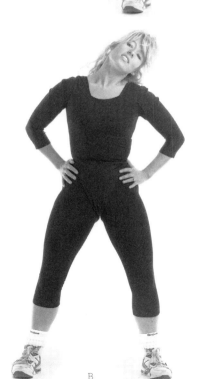

3. Shoulder Rolls

As you march on the spot, lift your shoulders to below your ears, the ears in line with the shoulder. Hold for the count of four, and then slowly pull them back down for four.
Reps: 8 for everyone.

B

WARM-UP

5. *Short Squats*

Starting Position:
Stand, feet together, knees soft, arms in front. Pay particular attention to the position of the knees in relation to the feet. If you remember how you walk and the position of your feet and knees as you walk, you can't go wrong.

Movement: 1. Lock your knees together and squat down until your thighs are parallel with the floor. (If the heels begin to rise from the floor, you've gone too far.)

2. From this half-way position, rise back up half-way to the starting position (as in photo), then down again. Keep the movement short and sweet.

Reps: 15 (beginners)
20 (intermediate)
25 (advanced)

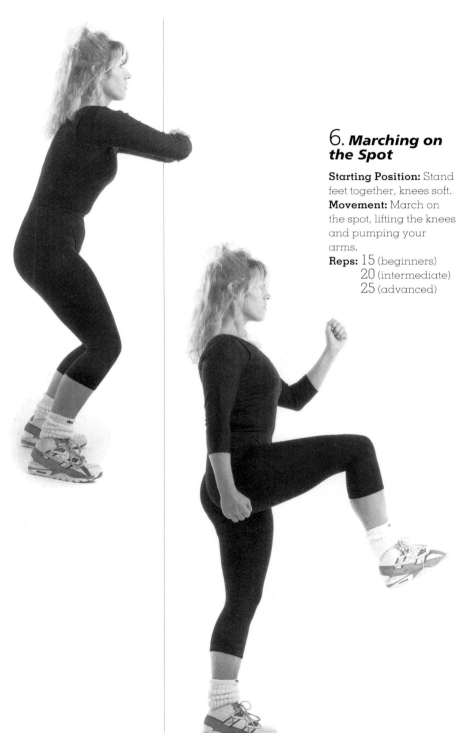

6. *Marching on the Spot*

Starting Position: Stand feet together, knees soft.
Movement: March on the spot, lifting the knees and pumping your arms.

Reps: 15 (beginners)
20 (intermediate)
25 (advanced)

WARM-UP

7. *Traffic Signal Squats*

Starting Position: Stand feet shoulder width apart, knees soft, hands lightly on shoulders.

Movement: 1. Bend knees slightly, raise both arms towards the ceiling (A), straighten knees but don't lock out, hands return to shoulders.

2. Bend knees, extend right arm out in front of chest, raise left arm up to ceiling (B), straighten knees, hands return to shoulders.

3. Bend knees, lift both arms towards the ceiling, straighten knees, hands return to shoulders.

4. Bend knees, extend left arm out in front of chest, raise right arm up to ceiling, straighten knees, hands return to shoulders.

Reps: Repeat whole sequence twice.

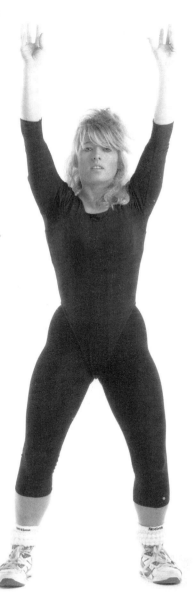

A

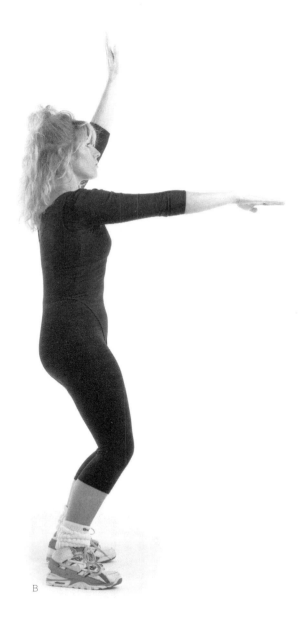

B

WARM-UP

8. *Side-Stepping Arm Scissors*

Starting Position: Stand, feet shoulder width apart, knees soft, hands on hips.

Movement: A stepping side-to-side movement.

1. Step right foot to left foot, then step right foot back into place.

2. Step left foot to right foot, then step left foot back into place.

3. Keep stepping side to side, then add your arms.

4. Lift both arms to scissor over head. Lower them and scissor over in front of waist.

Reps: 24 for everyone.

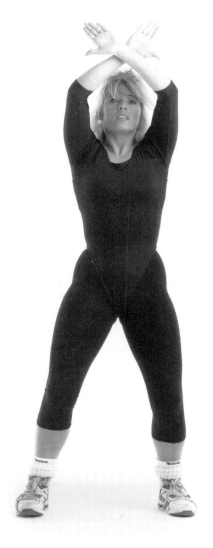

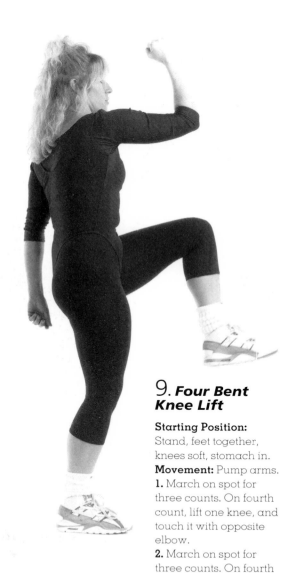

9. *Four Bent Knee Lift*

Starting Position: Stand, feet together, knees soft, stomach in.

Movement: Pump arms.

1. March on spot for three counts. On fourth count, lift one knee, and touch it with opposite elbow.

2. March on spot for three counts. On fourth count, lift other knee, and touch it with opposite elbow.

Reps: Repeat sequence 4 times.

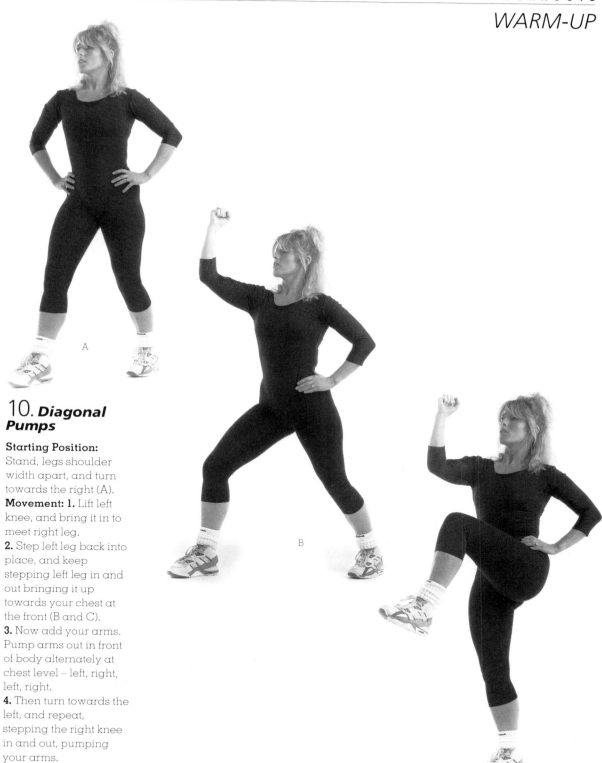

10. *Diagonal Pumps*

Starting Position:
Stand, legs shoulder width apart, and turn towards the right (A).

Movement: 1. Lift left knee, and bring it in to meet right leg.

2. Step left leg back into place, and keep stepping left leg in and out bringing it up towards your chest at the front (B and C).

3. Now add your arms. Pump arms out in front of body alternately at chest level – left, right, left, right.

4. Then turn towards the left, and repeat, stepping the right knee in and out, pumping your arms.

Reps: 16 on each side.

WARM-UP

11. *Grapevine*

Starting Position:
Stand, feet shoulder width apart, stomach in, hands out to the sides (A).
Movement: 1. Step to the side on the right foot.
2. Bring the left foot across behind the right foot, crossing arms in front (B).
3. Move the left foot back to starting position and bring the right foot behind the left.
Reps: 8 on each side.

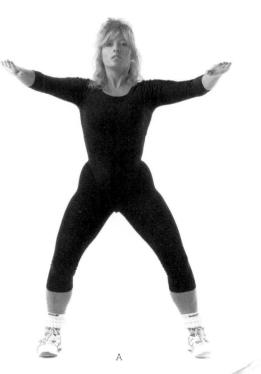

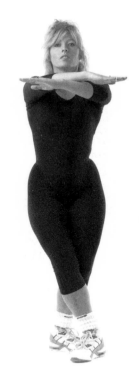

A   B

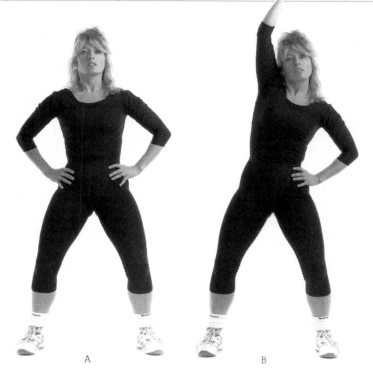

A   B

12. *Side Lifts*

Starting Position:
Stand, feet shoulder width apart, knees soft, stomach tight, hands on your hips (A).
Movement: 1. Bend your knees into a semi-squat and rise up with one arm towards the heavens (B).
2. Bend again and rise with the other arm extended. The opposite arm to the rising one should rest on the thigh.
3. Pay particular attention to back position; it should be directly over the hips. The movement should be flowing from one side to the other.
Rep: 16 on each side.

WARM-UP

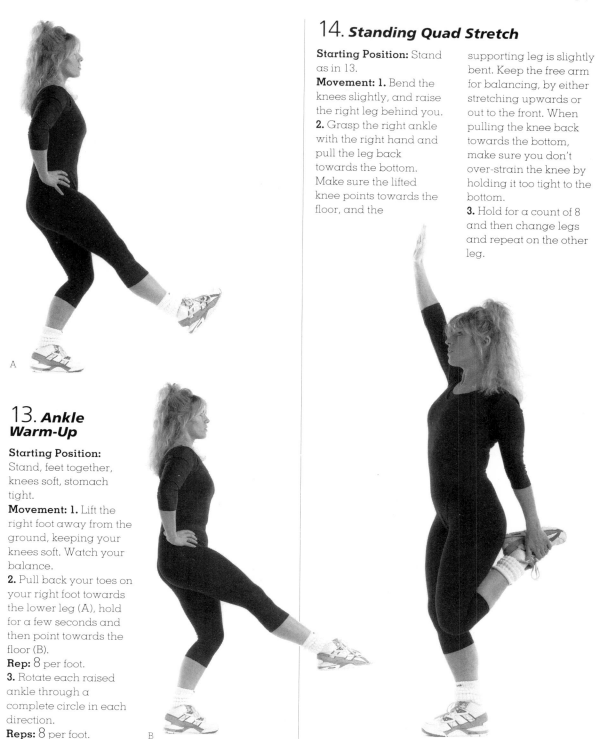

A

14. *Standing Quad Stretch*

Starting Position: Stand as in 13.

Movement: 1. Bend the knees slightly, and raise the right leg behind you.
2. Grasp the right ankle with the right hand and pull the leg back towards the bottom. Make sure the lifted knee points towards the floor, and the supporting leg is slightly bent. Keep the free arm for balancing, by either stretching upwards or out to the front. When pulling the knee back towards the bottom, make sure you don't over-strain the knee by holding it too tight to the bottom.
3. Hold for a count of 8 and then change legs and repeat on the other leg.

13. *Ankle Warm-Up*

Starting Position: Stand, feet together, knees soft, stomach tight.

Movement: 1. Lift the right foot away from the ground, keeping your knees soft. Watch your balance.
2. Pull back your toes on your right foot towards the lower leg (A), hold for a few seconds and then point towards the floor (B).
Rep: 8 per foot.
3. Rotate each raised ankle through a complete circle in each direction.
Reps: 8 per foot.

B

WARM-UP

15. *Inner Thigh Stretch*

Starting Position:
Stand, feet together, knees soft.

Movement: 1. Bend over with your right leg bent and the left leg extended out to the side.
2. Place your hands on your thighs. Under no circumstances, lock out the knee of the extended leg. Keep the head up and look forward throughout the whole motion.
3. Move the body from side to side, bending and extending legs, holding for the count of 8 on each side.

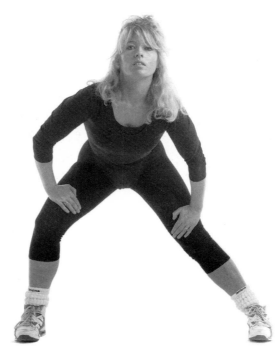

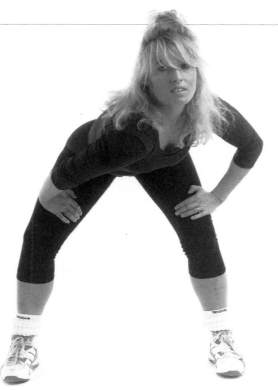

16. *Spinal Compression Relief*

Starting Position:
Standing, feet shoulder width apart, knees soft.

Movement: 1. Bend over and support the upper body by resting the hands on the thighs (the knees and lower leg should be at a 90° angle). The head should be kept up and looking forward.
2. Drop one shoulder towards the ground using the upper back only.
3. Hold for the count of 8 then do the other shoulder.

Reps: 4 on each side.

WARM-UP

17. *Lower Back Stretch*

Starting Position: Stand, feet together, knees soft.

Movement: 1. Lean forward and rest your hands on the knees, head up as for the previous exercise (A).

2. Slowly arch the back by sucking in the stomach muscles to tilt the pelvis under (a pelvic tilt) (B).

3. Hold for a count of 8 then release.

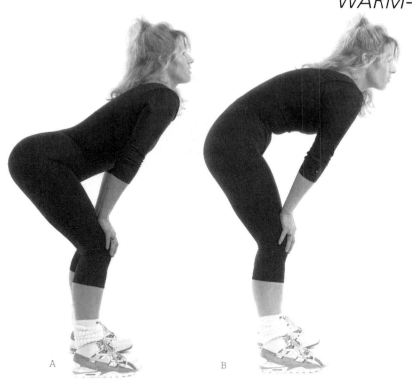

A

B

18. *Lunge*

Starting Position: Stand tall, feet and knees together.

Movement: 1. Step your left leg out in front and bend so that the thigh is parallel to the floor, with the right leg extended out behind. The front knee should be directly over the ankle but not beyond the toes.

2. Place your hands on your hips, and extend the back leg as far as possible behind you.

3. Push your hips towards the floor. Hold for a count of 8 on each side.

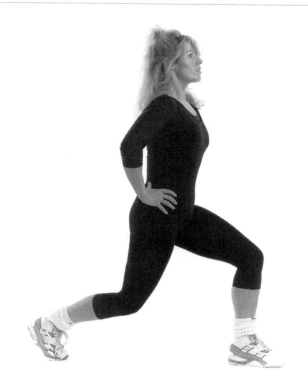

WARM-UP

19. *Hamstring Stretch*

Starting Position: Stand tall, then extend one leg out in front. Bend the other leg.

Movement: 1. Push your weight on to your back leg. Keep the knee soft and position the hands on the back-leg thigh.
2. Point the toes of the front foot up to the ceiling, and then press down for a count of 4.
3. Return to starting position and change legs.

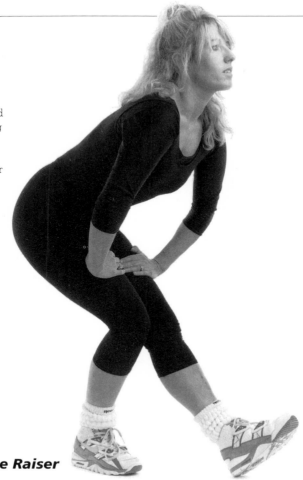

20. *Second Pulse Raiser*

This phase is designed to prepare you for the main aerobic circuit whilst bringing the pulse up to an aerobic level.

Start walking around the room, occasionally increasing the length of your stride. Curl your arms or pump your arms in the air above your head. Every so often, change the direction of the walk, to alter the forward stress. Break into a skipping motion, making sure you land with the knees soft. When you land, do so on heel then toe. Either place your hands on the hips or mimic a skipping motion with the hands. Start to increase the intensity of the exercise as you're about to attempt the big one.

To finish your warm-up, do a few of your favourite exercises (taken from the workout you're going to do on this particular day).

At this point, take your pulse to see where you are in the great scheme of things. Remember that your pre-exercise or resting heart rate can be anywhere from 50 onwards, but hopefully not much more than 80–90, depending on how fit you are. The average resting heart rate is approximately 72 beats per minute. During the first pulse raiser, the warm-up and the second pulse raiser, start to pick the pulse up, slowly bringing it up to your own fatburning level (65% of 220 minus your age). During the actual workout, try and maintain the pulse in your training range (65%–85% of 220 minus your age). If your pulse starts to creep over the top mark, slow yourself down by dropping the number of repetitions, or the speed at which you attack your workout. Remember, you should be able to hold a conversation at all times.

The Cool-Down

After you've pumped, jumped and worked your body to the max during your workouts, it's time to bring everything back down to earth again. The cool-down, like the warm-up, should be a controlled process, bringing you from the main workout back to your original pre-workout resting rate. (Don't get this mixed up with the *physical* state you started out with.)

Most people make the same mistake after they exercise. They stop dead in their tracks and wander off to the showers, sit down and in some cases, leap straight into the sauna. Big mistake on both counts. The body in all its wisdom has been directing blood during your workout to all the working muscles. Stopping abruptly can cause pooling of the blood in the muscles, thus starving the heart of blood. In most cases this makes you want to throw your guts up, and in some extreme cases causes you major grief with your ticker. If the ticker is a bit short of blood supply, this in due course will lead to a shortage of blood in the brain, and we don't want that. Most of us need all the movement we can get up there.

These symptoms can also be caused by a too hot bath, shower or a sauna. What you would be doing is exposing the body to increased heat at a time when it is trying to cool itself down. Also, as the body loses fluid during exercise, and this fluid loss would be continued during a sauna or steam bath especially, this could reach dehydration levels . . .

Hence cool-downs are an essential part of any workout, as the activity is designed to redirect blood flow back around the body, while taking the body back to its normal state of cool coma. Cool-downs should last long enough to do so, and they should include a static stretch at the end, while everything is still warm.

At the end of the whole thing, and you're in a state of post-exercise bliss, you should do your last pulse raiser. Just a minute or so of light activities to pick up the heart rate a few beats so you leave the world of exercise feeling on top of the world, not chilled out to the max, iceman.

At the end of the day, what the cool-down does is:
- Aids muscle relaxation.
- Removes build-up of lactic acids and waste produce from the muscles.

COOL-DOWN

- Reduces soreness of the muscles (but this is still debatable).
- Gives you a much deserved breather from the workout and generally signals the end of the class which has got to be good for all concerned.

Start your cool-down by reversing your warm-up, so instead of increasing your pulse you are bringing your pulse the other way, slowing down the movements. Work from page 66 back to page 56. All the exercises performed should be slow and deliberate with special attention paid to your breathing. All the stretch movements should be held for a count of 8. They should be taken past the normal range of motion, but always remember it's not 'no pain, no gain,' any more, but 'any pain, no train'.

Start by reversing the warm-up exercises, particularly the larger compound movements, and slow the tempo down as your breathing and body start to return to normal.

Then leap into the flexibility exercises on the following pages. When you've finished those, you might think it's all over for the day. Wrong. Just to finish it off, throw on your fav record or cd and throw a few funky moves around your training space to bring your pulse up a few beats, so you can exit your exercise mode with that loving feeling. Don't panic if you think you look like some demented Greek dancer. (If the truth be known, I couldn't throw anything resembling a dance move if you paid me.)

Well, that's the end of the story, but please don't forget, no *hot* water, and definitely no sauna. Try a moderate heat instead (it's not an excuse for doing without a shower, you stinky lot).

‘ Saunas result in weight loss that is only water loss. As soon as you drink, the water loss is replenished and the weight is regained. ’

COOL-DOWN

1. Back of the Arm

Starting Position: Keep at a slow steady walk around your exercise area.

Movement: 1. Touch your right hand to the back of your left shoulder, with the elbow pointing up to the ceiling. Bring the left arm over the top of the head and place on the elbow of the right arm.

2. Push down slightly on the elbow so that you feel the stretch in the back of arm. The shoulders should be pulled back.

3. Hold for a count of 8 and change arms.

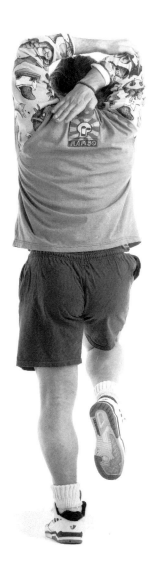

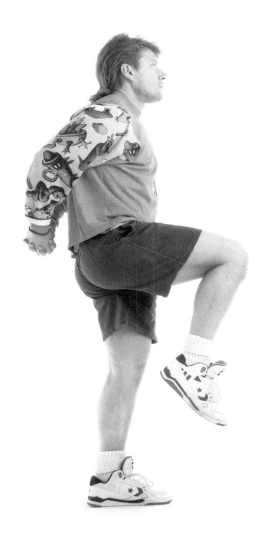

2. Chest Stretch

Starting Position: Still walking around the room.

Movement: 1. Bring your hands up behind your body, clasping them together with your elbows pointing upwards. The stretch should be felt in the front of the shoulders, sides of the chest and triceps. Particular care should be paid to keeping your head and body upright as you wander around.

2. Hold for a count of 8, release and then shake out the arms.

COOL-DOWN

3. *Neck Stretch*

Starting Position: Still walking.
Movement: 1. Tilt the head to one side, so you feel the stretch in the side of the neck and shoulder.
2. Hold for the count of 8 and then do the other side.

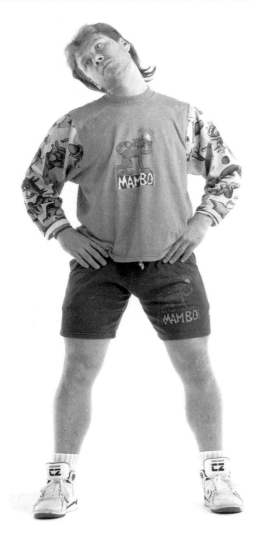

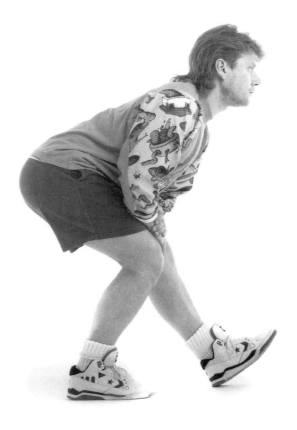

4. *Upright Hamstring Stretch*

Starting Position: Come to a grinding halt. Stand still and stagger the legs, supporting the hands on the thighs. The back leg should be slightly bent.

Movement: 1. Raise the toes of your front foot. The stretch should be felt in the back of the extended leg.
2. Hold the stretch for a count of 8 then change legs.

COOL-DOWN

5. *Calf Stretch*

Starting Position: Place yourself in a tee-pee position (bum high in the air, palms on floor).
Movement: 1. Keeping the heel of the left leg firmly on the ground, rest the right leg on the back of the left leg. The knee of the left leg should be kept slightly soft.
2. To make the stretch slightly easier, shorten the distance between the hands and leg. The stretch will be felt in the back of the leg.
3. Hold for a count of 8, and change legs.

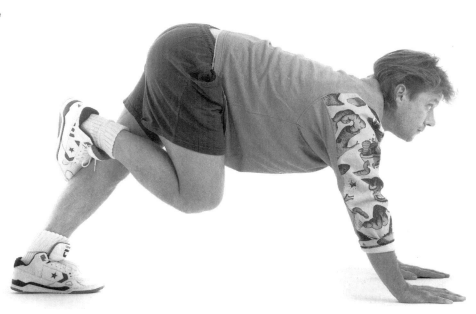

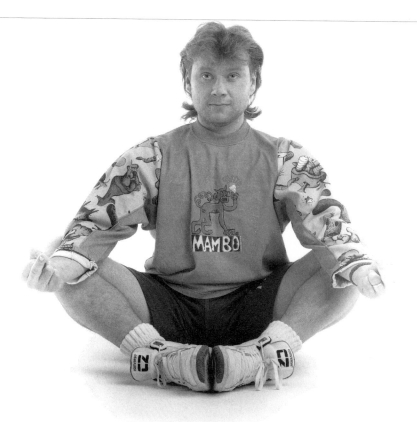

6. *Seated Inner Thigh Stretch*

Starting Position: Sit on your butt and place your feet together.
Movement: 1. Rest the elbows on the knees, lean forward with the body slightly and press down on the knees lightly with the elbows. The tension should be equal on both knees at all times throughout the motion.
2. Hold for a count of 8.

COOL-DOWN

7. Outer Thigh Stretch

Starting Position: Lie on your back.

Movement: 1. Extend both legs up from the body. Keep the right leg at a 90° angle over the extended left knee. Clasp the hands behind the extended thigh and pull both legs back towards the chest.
2. Hold for a count of 8 then change legs.

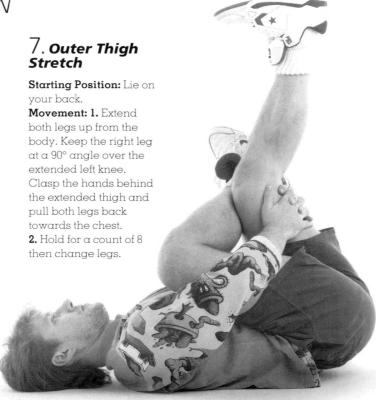

8. Hip and Back

Starting Position: Lie on your back, with the arms out to the side like a cross.

Movement: 1. Take the right knee across the extended left leg and gently push down. Try to keep the shoulders flat on the floor during the stretch.
2. Hold for a count of 8 and change sides.

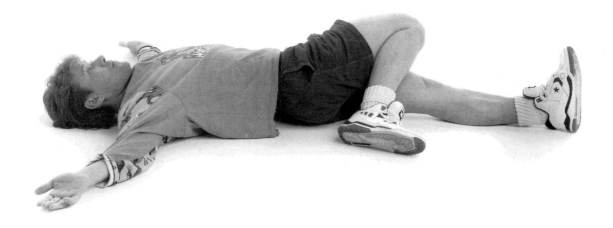

COOL-DOWN

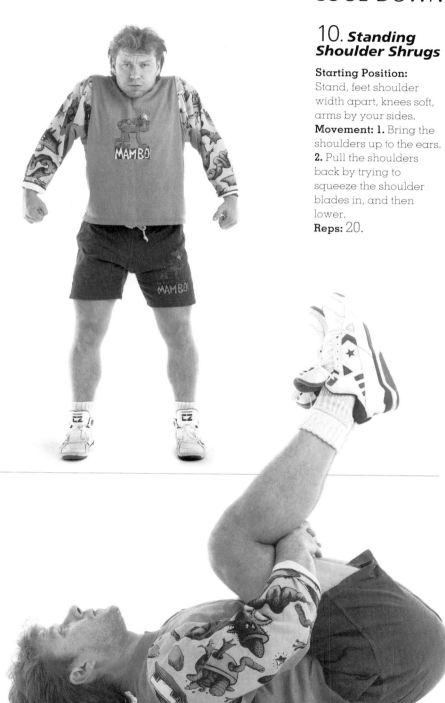

10. *Standing Shoulder Shrugs*

Starting Position:
Stand, feet shoulder
width apart, knees soft,
arms by your sides.
Movement: 1. Bring the
shoulders up to the ears.
2. Pull the shoulders
back by trying to
squeeze the shoulder
blades in, and then
lower.
Reps: 20.

9. *Lower Back Stretch*

Starting Position: Lie on
your back.
Movement: 1. Pull both
knees back to chest.
2. Clasp the hands
behind the thighs and
gently pull the thighs
towards the chest, at the
same time lifting your
bottom off the floor.
3. Hold the position for a
count of 8 and relax.

MONDAY'S WORKOUT

IN THE BEGINNING

A s we know, the secret of Fatbusting is not blowing a gasket on the workout, but low-intensity exercise. For exercise to be considered Fatbusting it must:

- Involve large groups of muscles, instead of the bed.
- Be continuous (excluding the warm-up and cool-down) for at least 15 minutes, at least three to five times per week.
- Be within your heart-rate training range (65–85% of 220 minus your age).
- Be low intensity. Breathlessness during your exercise programme would indicate that you are going too hard for an effective fat burn, and that you should slow down.

Start with once around the whole circuit, but as you get fitter in the next few weeks and feel that way inclined, try twice around. If you feel real daring you should be able to increase the circuit to three times around within the 30 days, without much of a problem. If you are still finding it easy, increase the amount of reps of each exercise, so instead of 15 try 20 etc.

Try not to stop between each individual exercise. You need to push as hard as possible, but always maintaining your pulse training range. (Remember 220 minus your age equals maximal heart rate: work at 65–85% of this.) Get into the habit of taking your pulse during your workouts, and if it's too high, slow down. Under no circumstances push to the point of pain. If you feel sick, dizzy or short of breath, cease exercising immediately.

Problems after Exercising?

When you start to exercise again, your body is going to complain. It will ache, it will get stiff, muscles sometimes cramp up and your joints make funny noises. Let's have a look at some of these problems, and try to sort out some of the anxieties related to losing your exercise virginity.

Muscle soreness

Muscle soreness is virtually impossible to avoid. There are basically three types of pain. The first is caused by the sudden increase in activity, but can be relieved by taking short rests during exercise. The second sneaks up on you one or two days later. All this means is that you're basically out of shape, and you've done too much. You've increased the intensity of your exercise too quickly; you should ease off the frequency, duration and intensity. Mild exercising will make it disappear in time. The third is caused by injury, a strain or a tear. If you suffer a muscle injury, the treatment will vary according to severity. For very mild strains, the best treatment is to keep using the muscle gently, slowly building up the intensity, and let the body do the rest.

Cramps

Cramps can be caused, like muscle soreness, by a sudden increase in activity, or by residual lactic acid deposits. Treatment is similar in both cases – continued activity, warm-up and cool-down, and static stretching of the cramped muscle. Lack of salt and fluids can also be responsible for cramps. If you perspire a lot, drink plenty of water, and use a small amount of salt with your food. When cramp strikes, do not use sudden, bouncing types of stretching, but stretch slowly and hold for a few minutes or until you can relax the muscle without it cramping again.

Creaky joints

Creaking and popping joints are a common occurrence. Don't worry, if there is no pain or discomfort, carry on exercising. The problem could be due to a lack of lubricating fluid in the joint, or it could be caused by the movement of tendons or ligaments over a bony protuberance as the joint bends. Make sure you warm-up properly: the heat created during warm-ups helps the joints move smoothly during exercise.

MONDAY

1. *Free-Standing Squats*

Starting Position:
Stand, legs shoulder width apart, knees soft, hands in front of you as in photo A.

Movement: 1. Gently squat down to the half-way position, making sure your heels never rise off the floor (B).

2. Return to the starting position. Do not bounce.

Reps: 15 (beginners)
        20 (intermediate)
        25 (advanced)

Note: Only bend knees slightly on straightening. Don't lock knees. Don't move hips

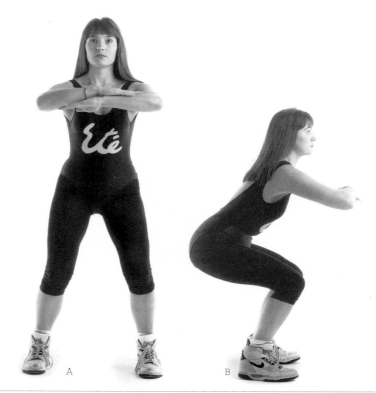

A   B

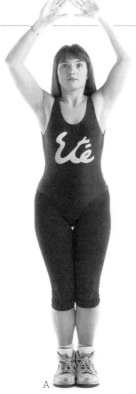

A

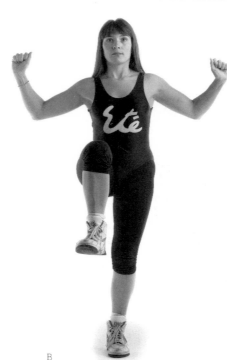

B

2. *Knee Lifts*

Starting Position:
Stand, feet together, knees soft, arms extended overhead (A).

Movement: 1. Swing your arms directly down towards your waist, and at the same time lift your right knee to the front of your body (B).

2. Repeat to the left-hand side. As you lift one leg make sure the other knee is slightly bent.

Reps: 8 per leg.

MONDAY

3. *Stride Jumps*

Starting Position:
Stand, feet together, knees soft, hands on hips (A).

Movement: 1. Keeping hands on hips and knees bent, jump both legs out and land shoulder width apart. Make sure when you land that your knees are kept soft, and feet are flat (B).

2. Return to starting position, and carry on.

Reps: 15 (beginners)
    20 (intermediate)
    25 (advanced)

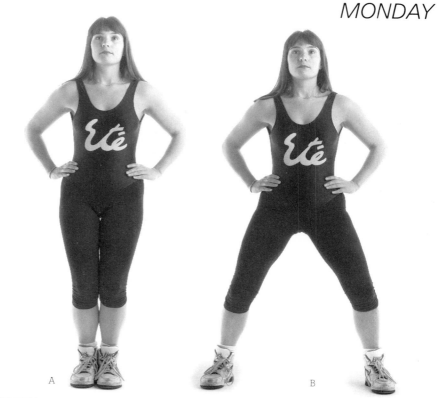

A   B

4. *Step Side Star Jumps*

Starting Position:
Stand, feet together, knees soft, hands by your side.

Movement: 1. Side step to the left. As you move your foot to the side, lift both arms straight out to the side, level to the shoulders, then return to starting position.

2. Do the same on the right-hand side, and then the left, right and so on.

Reps: 20 per side.

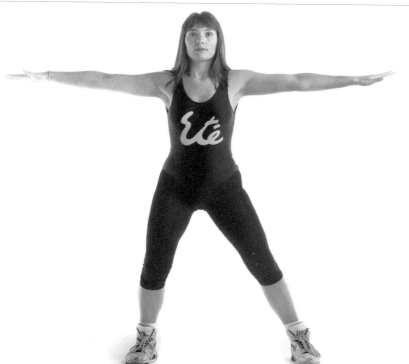

MONDAY

5. *Marching on the Spot*

Stand, feet together, stomach in tight, and march on the spot, lifting knees. Pump the arms to the top, and to the sides etc.
Reps: 16.

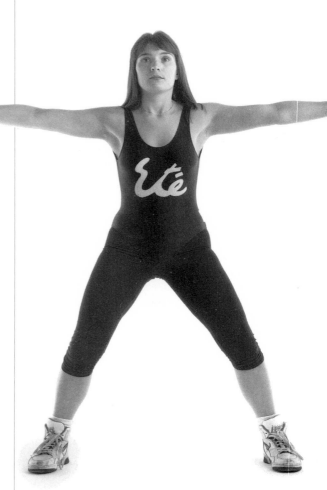

6. *High-Impact Star Jumps*

Starting Position: Stand, feet together, knees soft, hands on hips.
Movement: 1. Exactly the same as for a Stride Jump, excepting as you land, the arms should be fully extended to the sides, level with the shoulders. When you land, remember to keep the knees soft and land with flat feet.
2. Return to start position and start again.
Reps: 15 (beginners)
      20 (intermediate)
      25 (advanced)

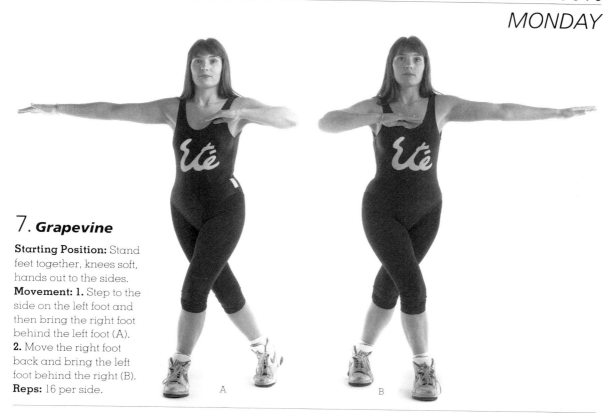

7. *Grapevine*

Starting Position: Stand feet together, knees soft, hands out to the sides.
Movement: 1. Step to the side on the left foot and then bring the right foot behind the left foot (A).
2. Move the right foot back and bring the left foot behind the right (B).
Reps: 16 per side.

8. *Box Press–Ups*

Starting Position: Kneel down on the floor on all fours. Make sure the hands are shoulder width apart, hands facing forward (A).
Movement: 1. Keeping your back straight, bend from the hips and lower your nose to the floor. Never lock out the elbows (B).
2. Return to the starting position. Keep the hands in line with the shoulders at all times.
Reps: 15 for everyone.

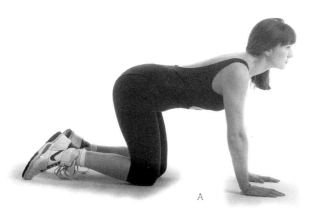

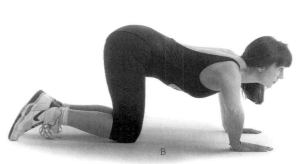

MONDAY

9. *Bench Dips*

Starting Position: Sit on a bench or chair. Place your hands facing forward on the edge of the bench or chair, shoulder width apart.

Movement: 1. Lift the body slightly away from the chair, feet in a box position to body, and the back as straight as possible (A).

2. Move the body down and up by bending the elbows out behind the body (B). Try not to raise the hips up at all during the movement, but use the arms always. Again remember not to lock out the elbows on the upward motion, and keep the back as straight as possible on the way down.

Reps: Try 8 to start with.

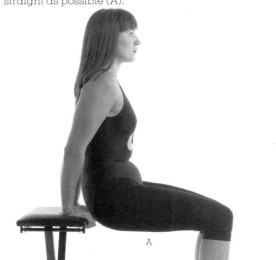

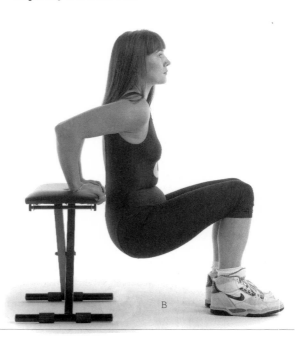

10. *Half Press-Ups*

Starting Position: Kneel on all fours as for Box Press-Ups (previous page) but keep the back in a straight line from shoulders to knees, and with the head up. Cross the ankles behind you (A).

Movement: Lower your nose to the floor, pivoting from the knees (B). Special attention should be paid to keeping the back straight as it will tend to sag. Again, don't lock out the elbows. And watch the hand placement.

Reps: 8 for everyone.

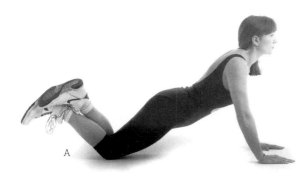

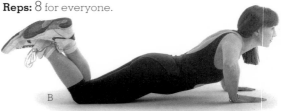

11. *Alternate Bicep Curls (with weights)*

Starting Position: Stand, feet shoulder width apart, knees soft. Hold the weights, and hang the arms down, palms forwards, keeping the elbows tight to your sides.

Movement: Lift the weights alternately upwards to the front, from waist to shoulder level keeping the wrists locked and straight through the whole motion, and the elbows tight to the sides.

Reps: 20 per side.

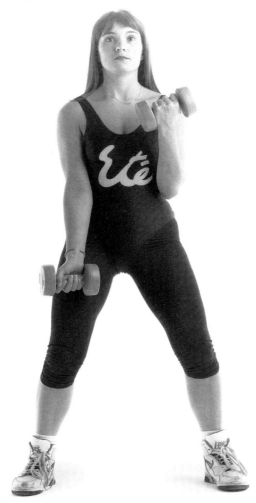

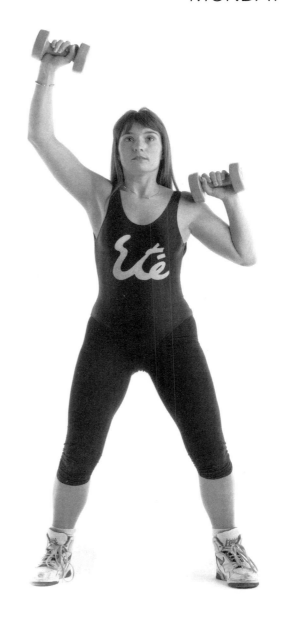

12. *Alternate Shoulder Press (with weights)*

Starting Position: Stand as at left. The weights rest at the shoulders, knuckles up and elbows down.

Movement: Raise the weights directly up from your shoulders and then back down to starting position. Again be careful not to lock out the elbows.

Reps: 20 per side.

MONDAY

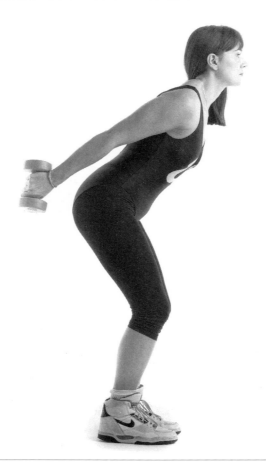

13. *Tricep Kickbacks (with weights)*

Starting Position: Stand, feet shoulder width apart, knees soft. Hold the weights down by your sides.

Movement: 1. Bend both arms back with your elbows pointing up to the ceiling. Knuckles facing the floor.

2. Without changing position, slowly straighten your forearms, without locking your elbows. The elbows stay still throughout.

3. Return to the starting position without bringing the elbows forward.

Reps: 15 (beginners)
20 (intermediate)
25 (advanced)

14. *Single-Legged Squat Thrusts*

Starting Position: Kneel down on the floor on all fours. Place the right leg straight out behind and tuck the left leg under the chest. Try and keep your head above the heart line (i.e. look straight ahead.)

Movement: 1. With a thrusting motion, change the legs, making sure the feet make contact with the floor. Keep the bottom down and the back straight throughout the motion.

2. Pay particular attention to hand placement throughout the exercise. The hands should be facing forward, elbows slightly soft and shoulder width apart. Under no circumstances, should the back sag during the exercise. The body should be tight and compact.

Reps: 10 per side to start with.

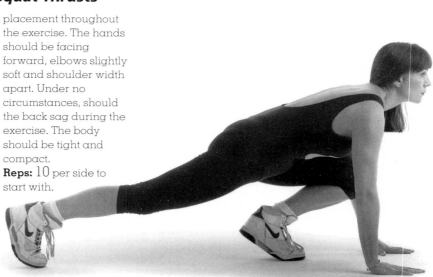

MONDAY

15. *Crunches*

Starting Position: Lie on your back, knees up, hip distance apart, ankles crossed.

Movement: 1. Frame the face with your hands and slowly lift your head and shoulders off the ground. Reach towards the knees.
2. Keep your back rounded throughout the exercise and try to keep your shoulder blades off the floor. Do not relax the muscles in your abdomen, and breathe regularly.
3. Return to starting position and continue.

Reps: 15 (beginners)
20 (intermediate)
25 (advanced)

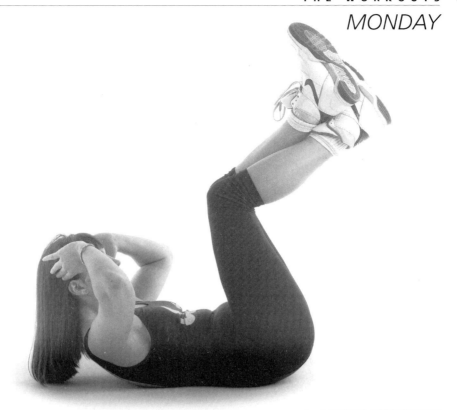

16. *Double Squat Thrusts*

Starting Position: Get down on all fours. The hands should be directly under the shoulders with the head facing forward.

Movement: Thrust both legs in and out simultaneously. Do not lock out the knees or let the back sag.

Reps: 15 (beginners)
20 (intermediate)
25 (advanced)

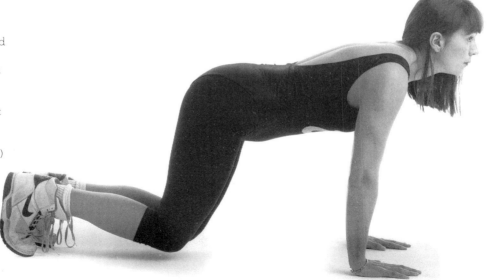

MONDAY

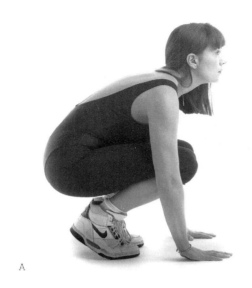

A

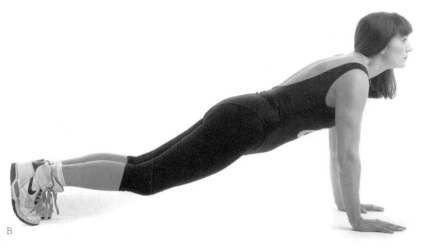

B

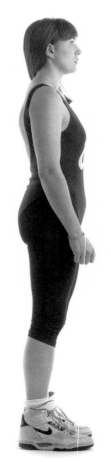

C

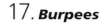

17. *Burpees*

Starting Position: Get down on all fours, then bring feet under hips (A).

Movement: 1. Thrust both legs out as in a Double Squat Thrust (B), bring them back under your hips, and then stand up straight (C).
2. Repeat the whole motion, and watch all the safety points of Single-Legged Squat Thrusts (on page 82).
Reps: 10 only, as this is a hard one.

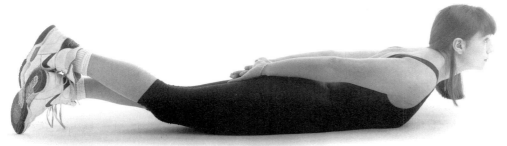

18. *Hyper-Extensions*

Starting Position: Lie on your stomach. Place your hands on your bum cheeks, and cross your ankles behind you. Make sure the hips are pressed firmly into the ground.

Movement: Slowly lift the upper torso away from the ground, without lifting the feet. The upper body only lifts from the hip area forward. Lift only as far as comfortable.

Rep: 15 (beginners)
     20 (intermediate)
     25 (advanced)

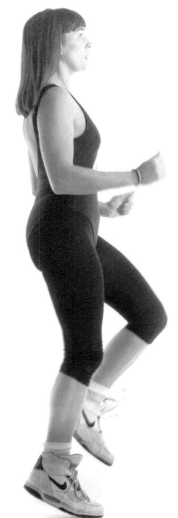

19. *Jogging on the Spot*

Stand feet together, stomach in. Jog on the spot, lifting your knees and pumping your arms. When you land, make sure you land on your heels then toes. Continue for 2–3 minutes to start with. Follow with some Marching on the Spot if you like.

Proceed into your cool-down phase immediately (see page 69) and thank God that's one day over.

TUESDAY'S WORKOUT

PUMP UP THE JAM

Gidday troops. Start with the warm-up you did yesterday, making sure that you're warm, sweaty and ready for today's workout.

This is entirely a weights workout, with a few circuit moves thrown in for good measure. If you're a total beginner, start with 15 of every exercise; if you consider yourself at an intermediate level, try 20 reps; and if you consider yourself a lean, mean, fighting machine try 25.

Basically, the weights workout has a whole body approach, with emphasis on large muscle groups. It might be an idea at this stage to dispel a few of the fallacies of weight training, and elaborate on a few home truths.

● Weight training adds bulk.

Weight training can result eventually in an increase of muscle size, though this increase varies with the individual, and the gender. The male sex hormone, testosterone, has a significant influence on the development of muscle size. The more of this hormone you possess, the more you will be predisposed to adding muscle size during a weight-lifting programme.

Women generally possess far less of this hormone, so therefore have a significant disadvantage in terms of increasing muscle mass during weight training. Any small gains which may result will be far smaller than that of men. Weight training for women, therefore, will generally tend to increase muscle tone and definition, rather than whack on the size.

● **Muscle-bound people are inflexible.**

If exercises are taken through the full range of motion then weight training will maintain or even increase flexibility rather than reduce it.

● **Speed decreases with strength gains.**

Research has shown that increases in strength tend to bring about increases in speed (Matthews and Fox, 1976).

● **Muscles turn to fat when you stop exercising.**

Muscles may get bigger, which is known as hypertrophy, when they are subjected to overload, and they may get smaller, atrophy, when they aren't worked. This process has little to do with fat accumulation which occurs when calories taken in exceed calories expended. If you stop exercising, your weight may go up if you continue to eat the same amount of food with a reduced energy expenditure. The fat stored has not been changed into slabs of muscles, although the fat may actually take up space that was once occupied by muscles.

● **Weight training is just for men.**

No way. In a health-related fitness context, the positive benefits of weight training can be applied to both men and women. From a cosmetic point of view, the benefits are just as applicable. From an ego point of view, men are still pissed off by women pumping weights, but I guess two out of three ain't bad. The majority of research in this area indicates that any exercise which is safe and effective for men is equally beneficial for women, with a notable exception being during pregnancy. Men can't quite get that trick together yet.

● **Does weight training make women monsters?**

In all my experience, women who weight train do it for one reason, and one reason only. Wait for it, not to bite the heads off chickens or show men up, but just because they want to look good. So when you decide to lift weights, questions will pop into your head like, will my excess fat turn into great slabs of muscles? But just think, next time you pick up a weight, of the shopping bags and babies you've carried around for years, therefore a 2.5 kg dumbbell ain't that heavy. As fat and muscles are two

TUESDAY

different types of cells, your stomach isn't going to turn into a huge bicep.

Even working out with light weights won't result in huge muscles. So, girls, shave your legs not your face, and keep on pumping iron, keep the reps high, and keep combining aerobic exercise with your weights programme, and always take a full-body approach to your workout.

Now let's plod on with the weights workout. Remember, to adopt the correct posture.

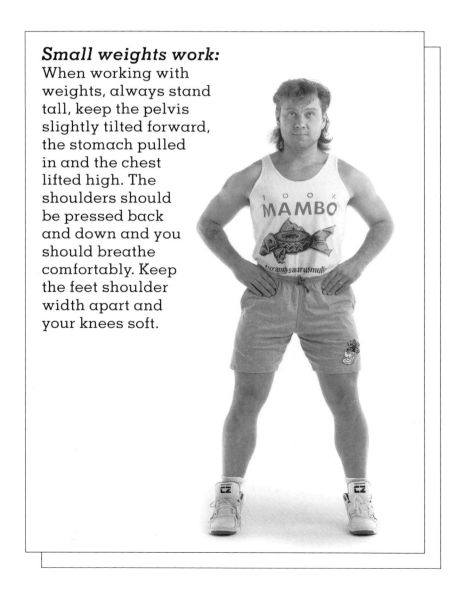

Small weights work:
When working with weights, always stand tall, keep the pelvis slightly tilted forward, the stomach pulled in and the chest lifted high. The shoulders should be pressed back and down and you should breathe comfortably. Keep the feet shoulder width apart and your knees soft.

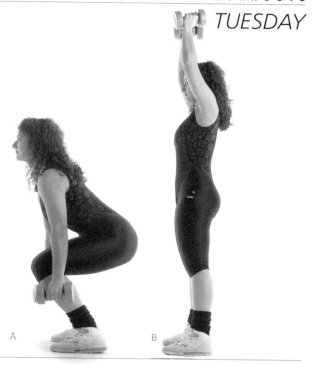

TUESDAY

1. *Half Squat and Press*

Starting Position: Stand, feet shoulder width apart, knees soft, weights held at the side of the body, facing down.

Movement: 1. Squat down, making sure your knees and thighs never go past the parallel position. Keep the back totally straight and slightly bent forward during the whole range of the exercise. Make sure the knees stay directly over feet throughout (A).

2. Squat slowly and return to starting position on completion of movement.

3. As you return to the standing position, bring the weights up the sides of the body to above the head, palms facing in and knuckles facing the ceiling. Do not lock out the elbows (B).

4. Return to starting position and commence the next one.

Reps: 15 (the unfit)
20 (the not so bad)
25 (trojans)

A   B

2. *Flying Laterals*

Starting Position:
Stand, feet together, knees soft, weights held at the sides of the body, knuckles outwards.

Movement: 1. Squat down slightly, keeping the knees tight and feet flat on the floor. As you squat down, place the weights directly under the knees (A).

2. Start to return to the starting position, and as you do, raise the weights from under the knees to level with the shoulders, in the shape of a cross. Keep the head upright, back straight and leaning slightly forward, and the elbows slightly bent (B).

3. Return to the squatting position with the weights under the knees and carry on.

Reps: 15 (beginners)
20 (intermediate)
25 (for the show-offs)

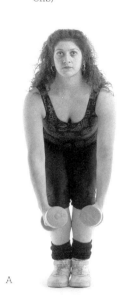

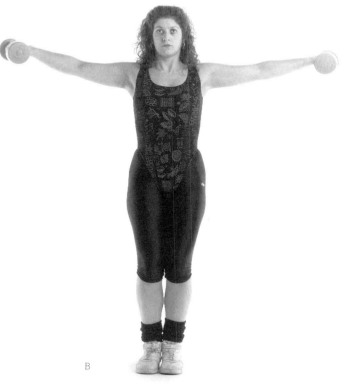

A   B

TUESDAY

3. Standing Calf Raises with a Press

Starting Position:
Stand, feet hip distance apart, knees soft, weights resting on the shoulders, knuckles facing the ceiling.
Movement: 1. Slowly rise up on your toes, so the heels leave the ground. As you lift up pump the weights towards the heavens, but yet again, don't lock out the elbows.
2. Return to starting position, by lowering the heels back to the floor.
Reps: 30 for everyone.

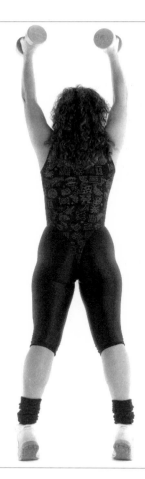

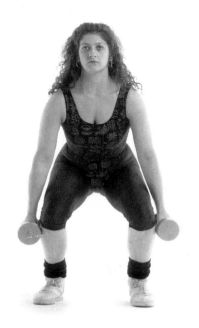

4. Half Squats

Starting Position: Stand feet and knees together, knees soft, weights held at the sides of the body.
Movement: 1. Squat slow and steady so that the knees and thighs are parallel with the floor. Hold your weights down to the side. Keep your head upright and looking straight ahead.
2. Squat down. If you find as you squat that your heels begin to rise up off the floor, squat only as deep as you can without the heels rising off the floor, even if it's only 6 inches (15 cm).
Reps: 15 (beginners)
      20 (intermediate)
      25 (advanced)

TUESDAY

5. *Stationary Lunges*

Starting Position: Stand, feet and knees together. Bend your left leg out in front, so that the thigh is parallel to the floor, and extend the back leg out behind, keeping the knee soft. Keep the head upright and looking forward, and watch out for an arched lower back. The weights are held on the hips.

Movement: 1. Squat up and down in this position, without letting the back knee touch the floor, or the front knee travel over the front foot.

2. After you finish one side, change legs.

Reps: 15 per side (beginners)
20 per side (intermediate)
25 per side (advanced)

Note: You could try some variations with the hand weights on this one, like curling or pumping the weights upwards or forwards.

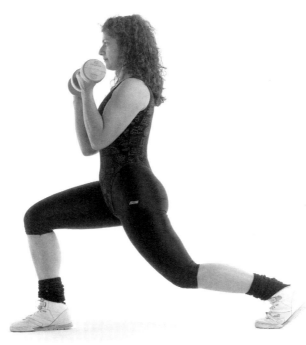

6. *Side Lunges*

Starting Position: Exactly the same as the stationary lunge, excepting this time you swing your legs to the sides, alternately.

Movement: 1. As you lunge to the side, return to starting position and lunge to the other side alternately.

2. As you lunge, curl the weights from hips to shoulders or press the weights from the shoulder upwards. Watch the elbow lock.

Reps: 15 per side for everyone.

TUESDAY

7. *Pre-Ski*

Starting Position: Stand, feet shoulder width apart, knees soft, weights hanging to the sides, with knuckles facing up.

Movement: 1. Exactly the same as the Half Squat, except your knees are apart, and this time as you squat, raise the weights up to shoulder level in front and back down as you lift up to starting position. Do not lock out the knees, so that you keep the resistance on the front of the thighs.

2. As you proceed, the arms and legs mimic a ski-ing motion.

Reps: 20 for everyone.

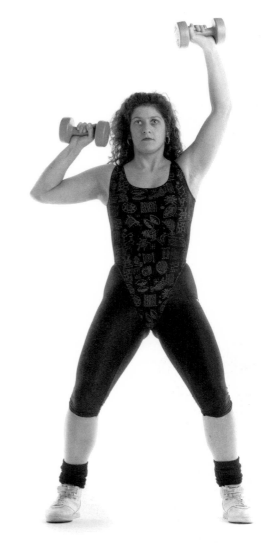

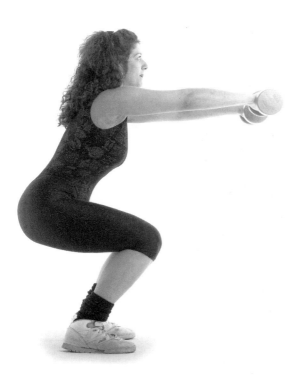

8. *Alternate Shoulder Press*

Starting Position: Stand, feet shoulder width apart, knees soft. Weights resting on the shoulders, knuckles facing back.

Movement: Keeping still, alternately raise one weight at a time. For variation pump both weights together, or jog on the spot pumping the weights. If you decide to jog remember to plant your heel on landing. Again, don't lock out the elbows, and keep control of the weights at all times.

Reps: 15 a side for everyone. If you jog, do so until you can't converse freely or whistle.

9. *Lateral Raises*

Starting Position: Stand, feet and knees together. Hold the weights in front of your crutch area, palms facing in and knuckles out (A).

Movement: 1. Slowly lift the weights sideways up to shoulder level, in the shape of a cross (B). Then back to starting position.

When the weights are at the topmost position, turn the thumbs down. Keep the elbows soft through the whole range of motion.

2. For variation, bend slightly at the knees, keeping the head and back in one straight line, and lift the weights frontwards straight out from the body, in the shape of a bent-over cross.

3. And for even more variation, as you perform lateral raises, move one foot at a time to the side, making sure you plant the heel and point toes up as you lift the weights.

Reps: 15 (beginners)
20 (intermediate)
25 (advanced)

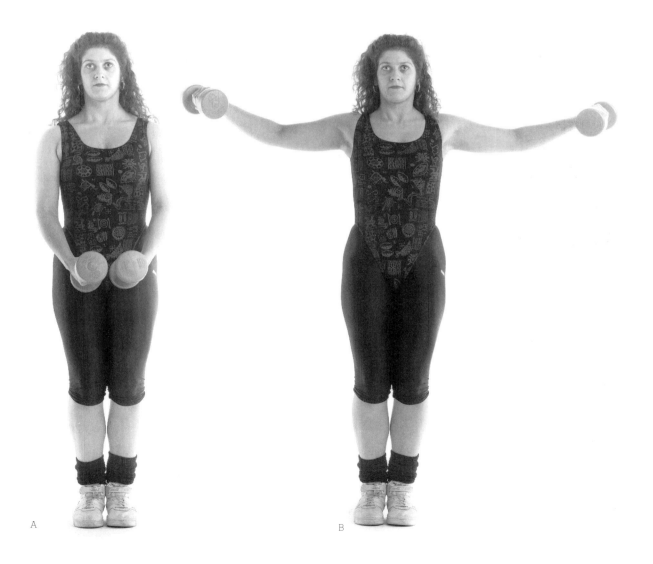

A   B

TUESDAY

10. *Alt Bicep and Head Curls*

Starting Position:
Stand, feet shoulder width apart, knees soft. The weights should be held at the sides, elbows tight into the sides and wrists locked. As you curl, the palms face up.

Movement: 1. For the Alt Bicep Curls, curl the weights alternately forwards and up to shoulder height, without moving the elbows from the hip area (A).

2. For the Head Curls, place the arms directly out to the sides in the form of a cross, palms up.

3. Curl the weights in towards the head and back again, without locking the elbows out. The arms stay at shoulder height entirely through out the whole motion (B).

Reps: Alt Bicep Curls: 20 each arm.
Head Curls: 20 each arm.

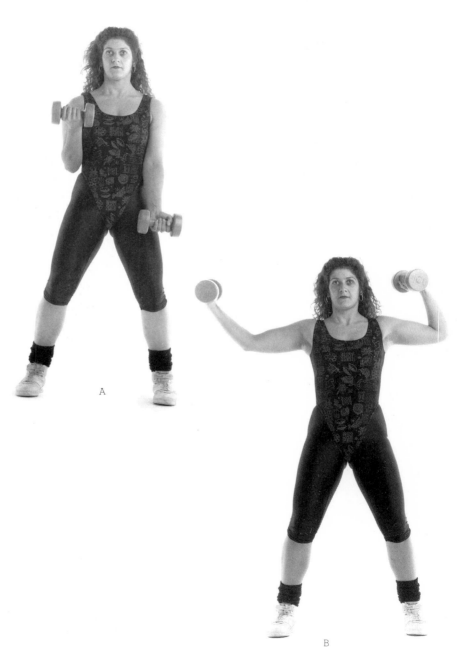

A

B

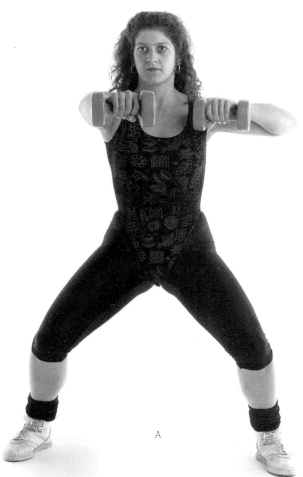

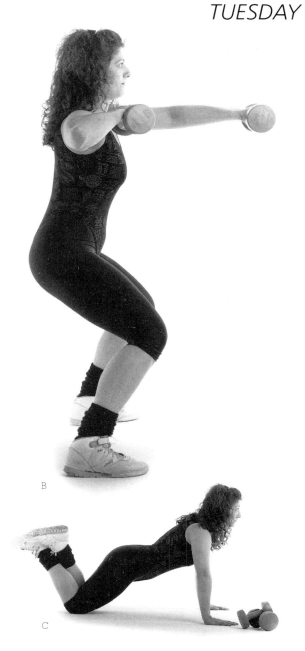

A

B

11. *Squat and Punch plus Half Press-Ups*

Starting Position: Stand, feet shoulder width apart, knees soft. Hold the weights directly out in front of you at shoulder level height, with the knuckles facing the ceiling.

Movement: 1. Squat down to the Half-Squat position and hold (A).

2. Slowly extend the arms out in a punch motion, one at a time. Make sure you don't lock out the elbows during the punches. Keep the head upright and breathe regularly (B).

3. As soon as you complete 20 punches each side, put the weights down, kneel and do a set of 20 half press-ups (described on page 80 in detail, but basically it's pivot from the knees to touch your nose to the floor (C and D).

Note: You could do box press-ups instead (see page 79).

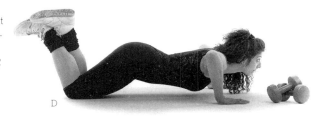

C

D

TUESDAY

12. *Tricep Chair Kickbacks*

Starting Position: Stand, feet together, knees soft, facing the chair or bench. Hold one weight in your left hand.

Movement: 1. Lean on the chair with your right hand.
2. Bend the left arm back, elbow to the ceiling.
3. Straighten your forearm without locking or moving the elbow.

Reps: 20.

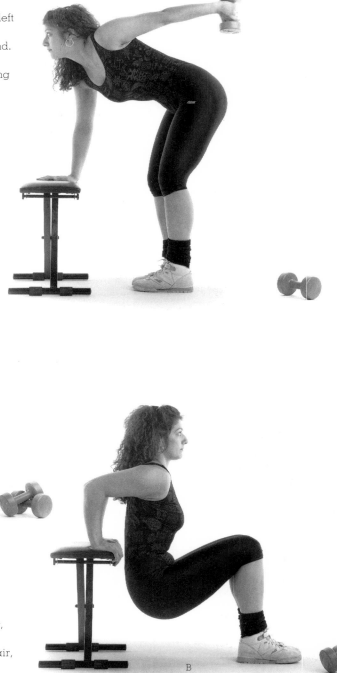

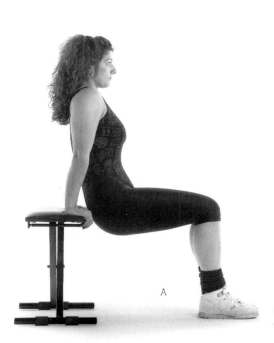

A

13. *Bench Dips*

Starting Position: Sit on the bench or chair. Place your hands facing forward on the edge of the chair, shoulder width apart (A).

Movement: Lift the body slightly away from the chair, by bending elbows out behind the body. Move the body down and up (see page 80 as well) (B).

Reps: 15.

B

TUESDAY

14. *Chest Flys*

Starting Position:
Stand, feet shoulder width apart, knees soft. Weights should be held out to the side of the body, in line with your ears, knuckles back. The elbows should be kept slightly soft through the whole range of the motion (A).

Movement: Curl the weights round in front of the body, as if giving someone a bear hug (B). Make sure you keep the line of the shoulders through the whole range of the motion.

Reps: 20 for everyone.

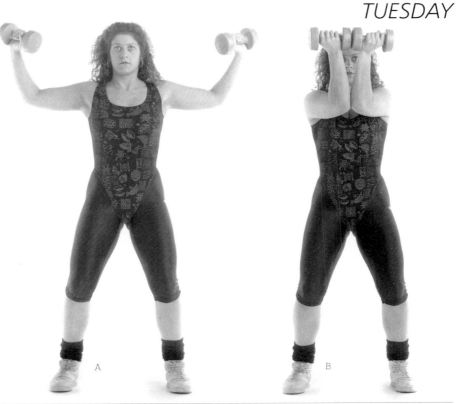

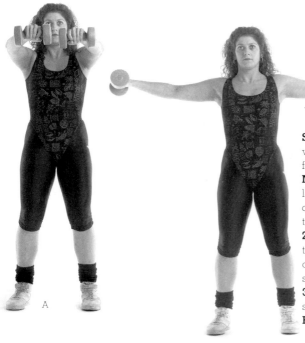

15. *Round the World with a Burpee*

Starting Position: Stand as above, except that the weights rest on the front of the thighs, knuckles forwards.

Movement: 1. First raise the weights, up to shoulder level in front on you (A), then out to the sides (like a cross) (B). Lower down to the sides of the body. Keep the arms straight, throughout the three movements.
2. After you've completed one Round the World, put the weights down and do a Burpee (overleaf: down on all fours, thrusting both legs out and in, then standing up straight).
3. Pick the weights up again and proceed with your set.

Reps: 5 (beginners)
     10 (intermediate)
     15 (advanced)

TUESDAY

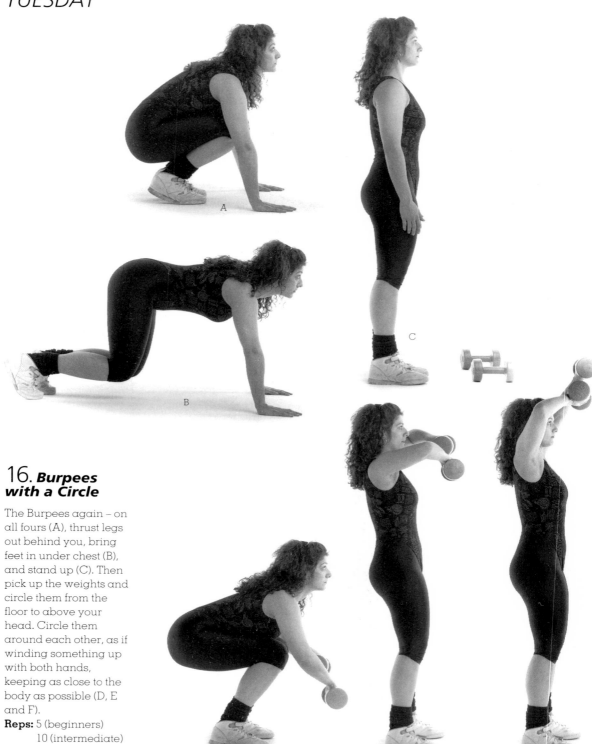

16. *Burpees with a Circle*

The Burpees again – on all fours (A), thrust legs out behind you, bring feet in under chest (B), and stand up (C). Then pick up the weights and circle them from the floor to above your head. Circle them around each other, as if winding something up with both hands, keeping as close to the body as possible (D, E and F).

Reps: 5 (beginners)
      10 (intermediate)
      15 (advanced)

TUESDAY

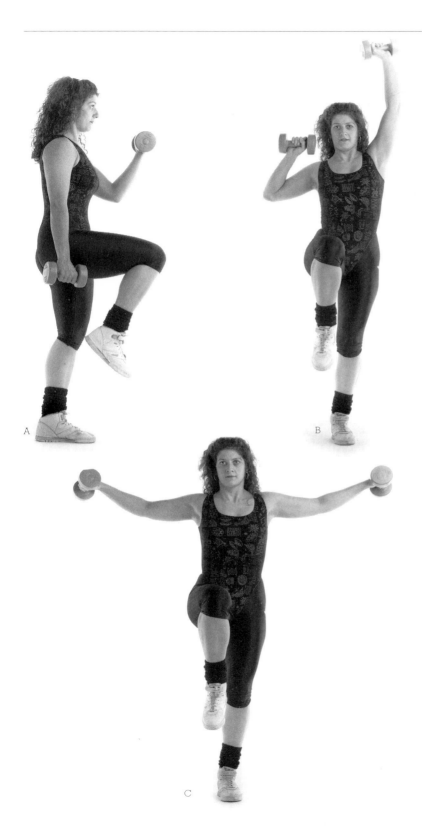

A

B

C

17. *Marching on the Spot, with Various Weights*

To finish off the workout, start marching on the spot, lifting your knees high and perform all the favourite weights movements that you have learned: eg raising alternately to shoulder height (A), above your head (B) or out to the side (C). Try a few reps of each. Remember to keep good form, even though you are marching on the spot.

Proceed straight to your cool–down, stretch and final pulse-raiser.

WEDNESDAY'S WORKOUT

TUMS AND NO BUMS

To achieve a firm stomach and waist – you know, the washboard effect – the muscles of the midsection must be strengthened. The term commonly used for the midsection is the 'abs' or *rectus abdominus*.

The stomach starts at your pubis and ends at the base of your ribs. The other group of muscles contained in this area is the obliques. They are generally mistaken for the side muscles, but these have very little value on a taut midsection. The external and internal obliques, however, make up the most part of a firm midsection, and therefore need to be worked accordingly. Unlike the rest of the body, you can exercise your obliques and abdominal muscles daily.

The other group of muscles that needs to be included is the muscles of the lower back, as these also contribute to a firm midsection via posture. Also, who wants love handles that extend from the side of the body to the back, a bit like a bum bag in reverse without the zip.

Hang on, some of you brighter dudes out there will be asking what's the point of just working out the midsection, as you can't spot-reduce a body area? You know that, and I know that, but it's a mind thing with most of us. Loads of tummy exercises have got to help slightly. I agree in a sense, because as you lose the body fat, there's got to be something lurking under there apart from your liver, kidneys and a pound of tripe. But being the kind of person I am, I've decided to throw in a few fat-burning nightmares to help along the fatburning process. So I'm sure that you

WEDNESDAY

will obtain the right pulse-training area with the right kind of push, and still keep working that stomach to the max.

Let's start, straight into the warm-up and on with the show. Take your pulse preceding the workout. And remember to adopt the correct posture for abdominal work (see page 54).

1. *Reverse Crunches*

Starting Position: Lie on your back, knees bent up, feet flat on the floor, hip distance apart. Place the hands under the buttocks.

Movement: 1. Cross the feet at the ankles and bring them up level to the hips.

2. From this position, bring the knees towards the chest, then return back to the hips. Never go past this position.

Reps: Try 2 sets of 10 to start with.

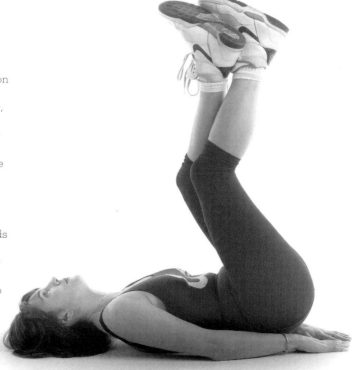

WEDNESDAY

2. *Diagonal Reaches*

Starting Position: Lie on your back, knees bent up, feet flat on the floor, hip distance apart. Hands behind or at the side of your head.
Movement: 1. Lift the head and upper back off the ground.
2. Reach across the body to the left knee with the right hand, then to the right knee with the left hand.
Reps: Try 20 a side.

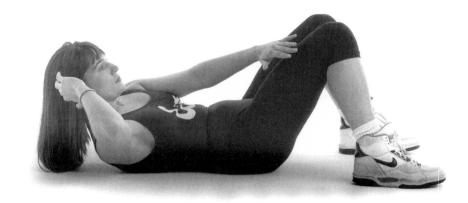

3. *Side Reaches*

Starting Position: Lie on your back, knees bent up, feet flat on the floor, hip distance apart.
Movement: 1. Lift the shoulders and head up from the floor.
2. Put one hand by your head, and the other by your side. Reach alternately towards one foot then the other. The arm slides down the side of the body trying to touch the foot (A and B).
Reps: Try 15 a side.

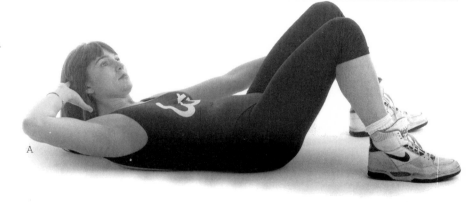

A

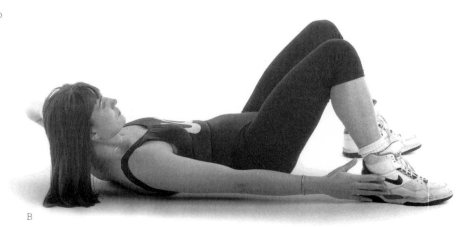

B

WEDNESDAY

4. *Tight Crunches*

Starting Position: Lie on your back, knees bent up, feet flat on the floor, hip distance apart.
Movement: 1. Bring the knees up and above the hips with the feet crossed at the ankles. The thighs and lower leg should be at a 90° angle to the body.
2. Place the hands by the sides of the head with the elbows pointing forward.
3. Slowly curl the head and shoulders towards the knees, trying to touch the knees with the elbows. Keep the whole motion tight at all times.
Reps: Try a set of 15.

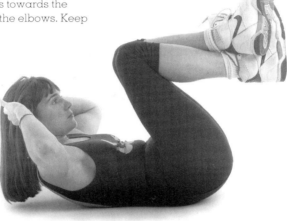

5. *Pelvic Tilt with Bum Squeezes*

Starting Position: Lie on your back, knees bent up, feet flat on the floor, hip distance apart.
Movement: 1. Tilt your pelvis so that your bum comes slightly off the floor.
2. Hold in the position, and squeeze the cheeks of your bum in for a count of 4 then release.
3. Lower back to the floor.
Reps: 10 for everyone.

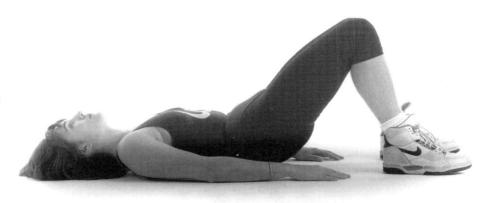

WEDNESDAY

6. *Hyper-Extensions*

Starting Position: Lie on your stomach, place your hands on your bum cheeks, and cross your ankles behind you.

Movement: 1. Lift your upper body from the hips. All the pressure should be felt in stomach, hips and lower back.

2. Keep the position for 30 seconds, then release.

Reps: 20 for everyone.

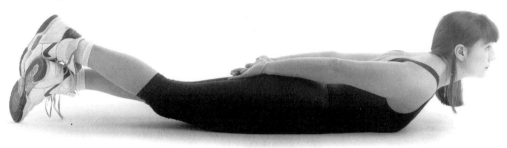

7. *Single-Legged Squat Thrusts*

Starting Position: Kneel down on the floor on all fours. Place the right leg straight out behind and tuck the left leg under the chest. Try and keep your head above the heart line (i.e. look straight ahead.)

Movement: 1. With a thrusting motion, change the legs, making sure the feet make contact with the floor. Keep the bottom down and the back straight throughout the motion.

2. Pay particular attention to hand placement throughout the exercise. The hands should be facing forward, elbows slightly soft and shoulder width apart. Under no circumstances, should the back sag during the exercise. The body should be tight and compact.

Reps: 20 per leg.

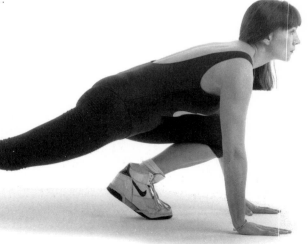

WEDNESDAY

8. *Double Squat Thrusts*

Starting Position: Get down on all fours. The hands should be directly under the shoulders with the head facing forward.
Movement: Thrust both legs in and out simultaneously. Do not lock out the knees or let the back sag.
Reps: 15 for everyone.

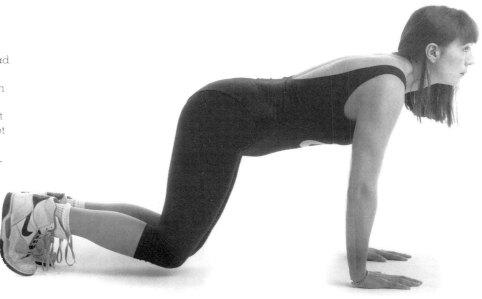

9. *Hyper-Extensions*

As for Exercise 6 opposite.
Reps: 20 for everyone.

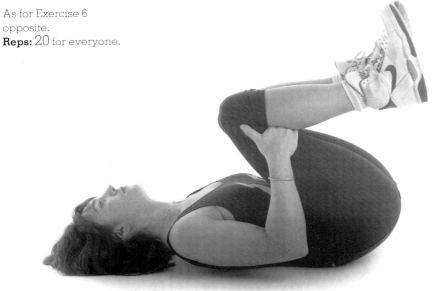

10. *Floor Back Stretch*

Starting Position: Lie on your back, knees bent up, feet flat on the floor, hip distance apart.
Movement: 1. Bring both knees up towards the chest.
2. Link your hands behind the thighs, and pull the thighs towards the chest, lifting your bottom off the floor.
3. Hold for a count of 8 and relax.

WEDNESDAY

11. *Crunch and Extend the Legs*

Starting Position: Lie on your back, knees bent up, feet flat on the floor, hip distance apart, hands by the sides of the head, elbows pointing forward.

Movement: 1. Bring the knees up over your chest, ankles crossed (A).

2. Curl your upper body up towards the knees.

3. As you do, extend the legs from the 90° angle straight up towards the ceiling. The upper body and legs should form a staple shape. When the legs are fully extended up they should be directly over the hips (B).

Reps: 10 for everyone.

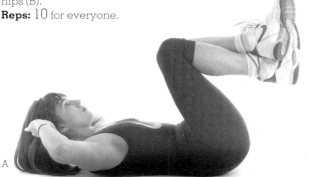
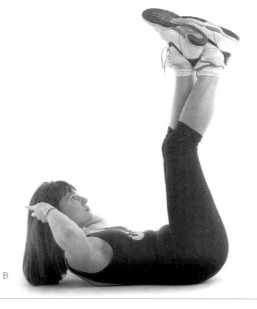

A

B

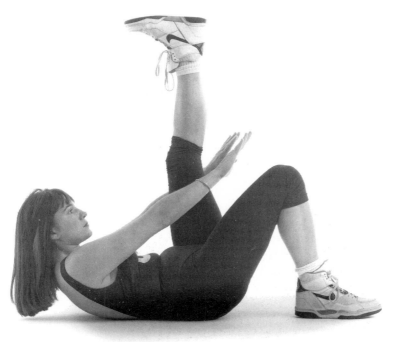

12. *Abdominal Pushes*

Starting Position: Lie on your back, knees bent up, feet flat on the floor, hip distance apart.

Movement: 1. Raise your left leg straight up towards the ceiling, and place your hands on either side of the extended leg.

2. As you lift the upper back and shoulders off the ground, push the hands forward and away from the knee.

Reps: Try 15 on this side, and then change legs for another 15.

13. *Jack Knives*

Starting Position: Lie on your back, knees bent up, feet flat on the floor, hip distance apart.

Movement: 1. Lift both legs up towards the ceiling and cross them at the ankles. The legs should be directly over the hips and the knees kept slightly bent.

2. Reach up with your left hand and touch the right foot (A) and then the right hand to the left foot (B). When you lift, only lift the upper back and shoulder off the ground.

Reps: Try 15 per side.

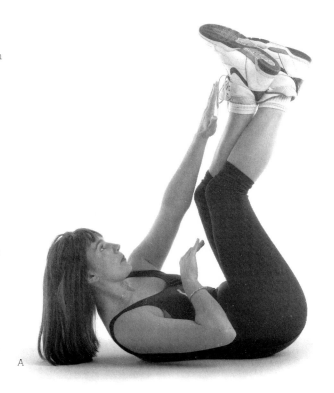

A

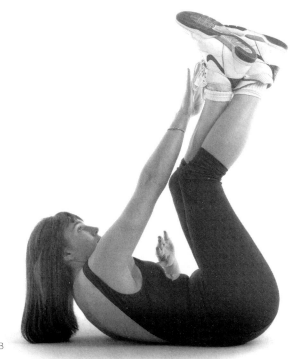

B

WEDNESDAY

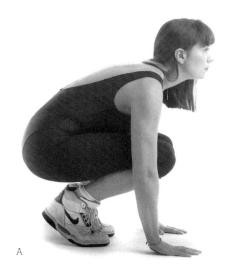

A

14. *Burpees*

Starting Position: Get down on all fours, then bring feet under hips (A).

Movement: 1. Thrust both legs out as in a Double Squat Thrust (B), bring them back under your hips, and then stand up straight (C).

2. Repeat the whole motion, and watch all the safety points of Single-Legged Squat Thrusts (see page 82).

Reps: 15 for everyone.

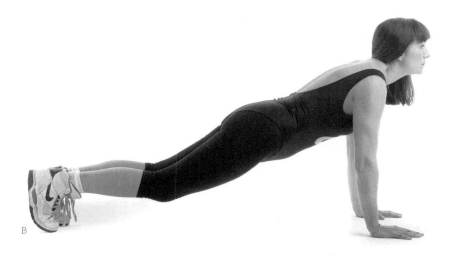

B

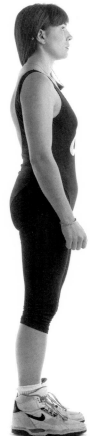

C

WEDNESDAY

15. *Stride Jumps*

Starting Position: Stand, feet together, knees soft, hands on hips (A).

Movement: 1. Keeping hands on hips and knees bent, jump both legs out and land shoulder width apart. Make sure when you land that your knees are kept soft, and feet are flat (B).

2. Return to starting position, and carry on.

Reps: 25 for everyone.

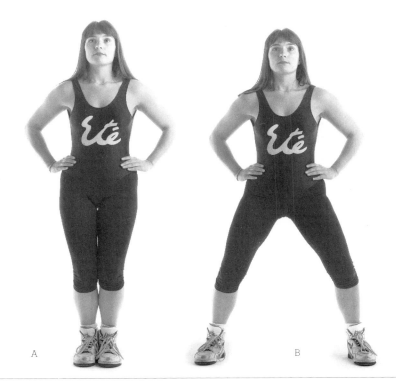

A   B

16. *Standing Side Bends*

Starting Position: Stand, feet shoulder width apart, knees soft.

Movement: Reach down the right-hand side of the body with the right arm and then down the left–hand side with the left hand.

Reps: 20 per side, alternating.

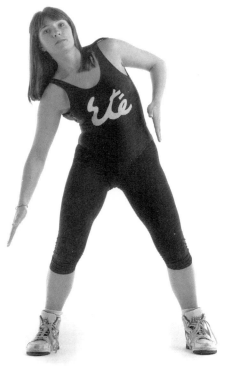

WEDNESDAY

17. *Half Press-Ups*

Starting Position: Kneel on all fours, then straighten back in a line from shoulders to knees, and keep the head up. Cross the ankles behind you (A).

Movement: Lower your nose to the floor, pivoting from the knees. Special attention should be paid to keeping the back straight as it will tend to sag (B). Again, don't lock out the elbows. And watch the hand placement.

Reps: 15 for everyone.

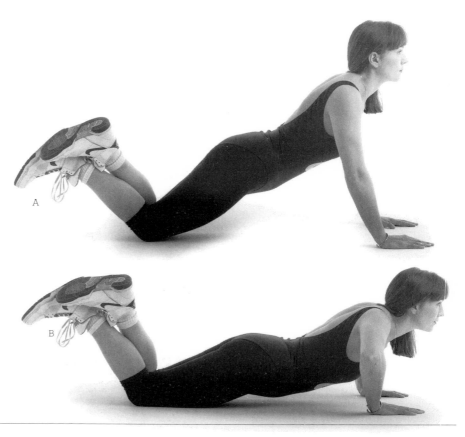

18. *Short Ab Curls*

Starting Position: Lie on your back, feet flat on the floor, hip distance apart. The hands should be around the side of the face.

Movement: Slowly lift your head and shoulders off the floor. As you rise, look to the ceiling. This movement is very small and concentrated.

Reps: 2 sets of 10.

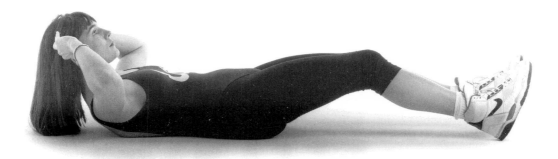

WEDNESDAY

19. *Torso Stretch*

Starting Position: Sit on the floor and cross your ankles in front of you. Place your right hand on the floor close to your hips. The arm must be kept slightly bent (but no elbow lock).

Movement: 1. Bring your left arm up and over your head in line with your shoulders.
2. Slowly lift the upper body up and across to the side of the supporting arm.
3. Hold for 30 seconds then change sides.

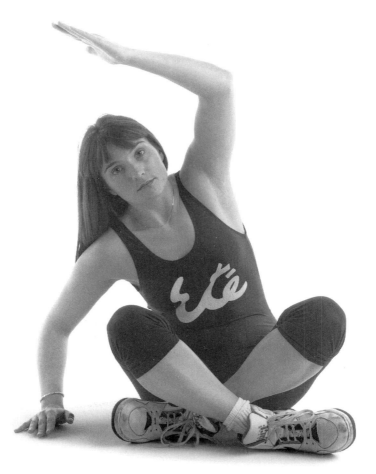

Take your pulse, making sure you're still in your pulse-training range, and then proceed straight into the cool-down. Don't forget to finish off the class with the final pulse raiser before you call it a day. Progression is a tricky one with the tum because you don't want to be sitting there doing hundreds and hundreds of sit-ups. I've found that with abdominal workouts it's not the number of reps but the *form*. So may the form be with you, and the stomach workout sufficient for the length of the course. The other bits that keep your pulse in the right area (for instance, Squat Thrusts, Press-Ups and Stride Jumps etc) can be increased accordingly as your level of fitness increases.

Catch you in the next workout – same time, same channel, different strokes for different folks – when we 'bash the bum' amongst other things. A thought to bear in mind, there's only two days to go this week, quickly followed by five weeks, and then not so quickly by three score and ten years . . .

THURSDAY'S WORKOUT

THE LOWER HALF

The legs and bum don't need much explaining, apart from the fact that they hold your upper body up, and are usually the bits you hate the most. The legs play a major part in your weight-loss programme, as one of the major factors in a good fat-burning programme is using large groups of muscles. It's also the upper legs and bum that win hands down in the size game, especially those afflicted with what is known as cellulite.

Does it or doesn't it exist? Personally, I think cellulite is a nasty way to describe fat. A word that conjures up maximum fear in all women worldwide. Forget the orange-peel thighs, mention this word and a woman turns to blancmange.

I don't dispute the existence of a *different* form of fat around women's thighs (or, more to the point, the girdle area), but fat it is, and if it's fat it can be removed, like all other fat on the body, through exercise and a good eating plan.

Cellulite has been researched fairly thoroughly, and various factors have emerged.

- It has a dimpled look, while ordinary fat has a fat look.
- It generally feels colder than other deposits of fat, suggesting that you're probably dead. The cold feeling is most likely due to bad circulation in this area. Interestingly, women who have cellulite and sit down all day generally have the worst deposit where the legs meet the edge of the chair, the place where the circulation is cut off the most.

THURSDAY

- Cellulite is not just an older women's problem. It can be found in extremely young girls, which leads to the theory that cellulite is caused by the presence of oestrogen: the more oestrogen present, the more chance of developing the lurgie.
- The danger times are puberty, pregnancy, menopause (although this means *less* oestrogen, it also means a slowing down of metabolism), and periods of stress.

Most recent research suggests that this special form of fat is caused by water retention due to toxins in the body. For some reason, some fat cells hold far more toxins than others, which in turn leads to the body surrounding these toxins with fluid, causing a waterlogged effect. Lifestyle plays a major part in this complaint. There is plenty of evidence to suggest that poor nutrition, stress, drugs, lack of exercise, stimulants such as alcohol, cigarettes, tea, coffee and chocolate, poor circulation, and a sluggish system, can all contribute to toxin retention and thus to cellulite. All these classical bad things are associated with an unhealthy lifestyle that someone interested in a fitness regime would slowly drop.

So can I cure cellulite? Yes, I think that the answer to this worldwide bane of women is exercise and a good healthy lifestyle. The programmes in this book will all, slowly but steadily, work on the three major aspects of the problem. Exercise, particularly of the areas affected, will improve the circulation and bump up the body's system to the max, therefore making the body far more efficient at removing toxins. Secondly, the exercise programmes will instil a desire to improve the lifestyle habits which are related to the production of toxins. Finally, exercise and good eating habits will generally lead to less fluid retention and the ability to burn fat more effectively than ever before.

Cellulite *can* be whittled away before your eyes, without having to wrap your thighs in seaweed, put 250 volts regularly through your legs, or immerse yourself in mud up to your eyeballs!

But now, let's get on with it, straight into the warm-up and then on to the workout. It's thigh and gutbusting time. Remember posture – although you should know it all by now.

THURSDAY

1. *Free-Standing Squats*

Starting Position:
Stand, feet shoulder width apart, knees soft, hands on hips.
Movement: 1. Gently squat down to the half–way position, making sure your heels stay on the ground during the whole movement.
2. Return to the starting position.
Reps: 15 (beginners)
　　　 20 (intermediate)
　　　 25 (advanced)

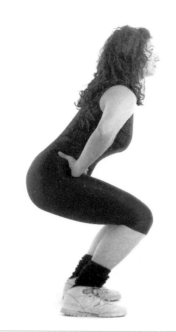

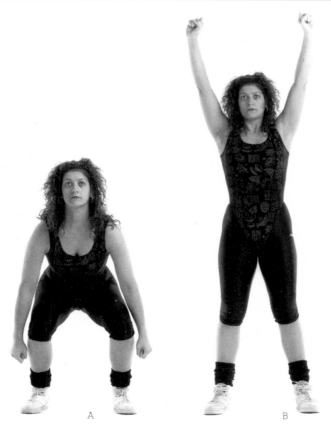

A   B

2. *Squat and Reach*

Starting Position:
Exactly the same as for the Free-Standing Squat, but hands by your sides.
Movement: As you squat (A), touch the floor with your hands, then reach up towards the ceiling as you extend up (B). Clench the hands.
Reps: 15 (beginners)
　　　 20 (intermediate)
　　　 25 (advanced)

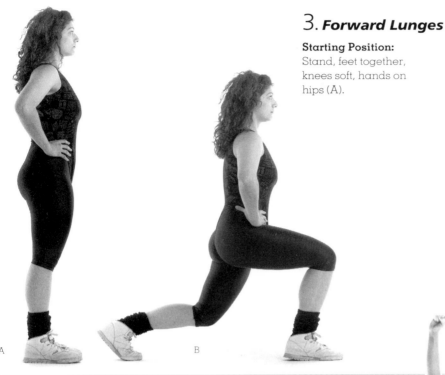

A   B

3. **Forward Lunges**

Starting Position:
Stand, feet together, knees soft, hands on hips (A).

Movement: 1. Step out with the right leg bent to form a 90° angle with the right thigh and knee. The left leg should be extended out behind with the heel facing the ceiling. Watch for lower back arch (B).
2. Return to starting position and step out with the left leg. The stepping should always be forward.
Reps: 15 each side, alternately.

4. **Tuck Jumps**

Starting Position:
Stand, feet shoulder width apart, knees soft.
Movement: 1. Squat down, keeping thighs parallel to the floor, and hands close together between the feet. Use the thighs to reach down, don't just lean forward. Watch the same safety points as Half Squats (see page 90) (A).
2. Jump and lift your hands above your head at the same time (B). Remember to keep your knees soft on landing.

3. Return to the Half-Squat position, with your hands between your feet, and carry on.
Reps: 25 for everyone.

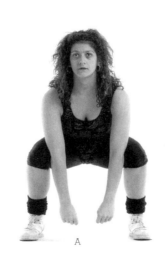

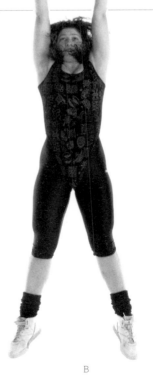

A   B

THURSDAY

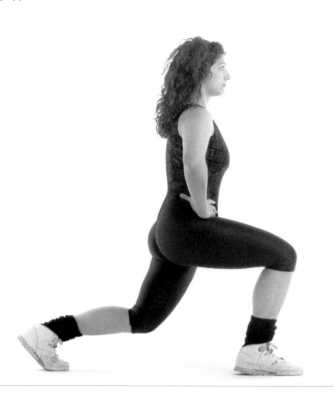

5. *Stationary Lunges*

Starting Position: Stand, feet together, knees soft, hands on hips.

Movement: 1. Step out exactly as you would for a Forward Lunge.
2. Stay in this position, and gently squat up and down, and then change sides and do the same on the other leg. Care should be taken that the knee of the back leg never goes near the floor, and that the knee of the front leg doesn't travel over the front foot. Keep the head upright and back straight throughout the exercise.
Reps: 16 per leg.

6. *Skip and Tuck Jumps*

Starting Position: Half squat down with the feet together and the hands under the knees. The head should be up and the back straight and slightly forward of the hips (A).

Movement: 1. Jump the feet out to shoulder width apart, making sure you land flat-footed and with the knees bent slightly. The hands come up level to the top of the shoulders, either forward of the body or to the sides of the body (B).
2. Return to the starting position and start again.
Reps: 25 for everyone.

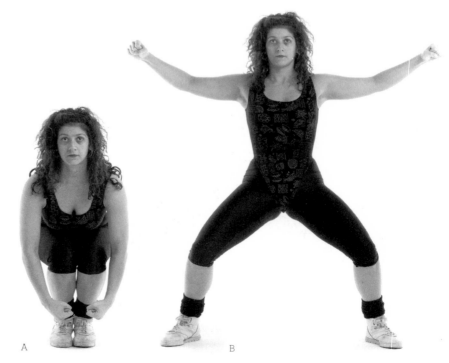

A

B

THURSDAY

7. *Pre-Ski*

Starting Position:
Stand, feet shoulder width apart, knees soft, arms hanging to the sides.

Movement: 1. Exactly the same as the Half Squat, except your knees are apart, and this time as you squat, raise your arms up to shoulder level in front and back down as you lift up to starting position. Do not lock out the knees, so that you keep the resistance on the front of the thighs.

2. As you proceed, the arms and legs mimic a ski-ing motion.

Reps: 25 for everyone.

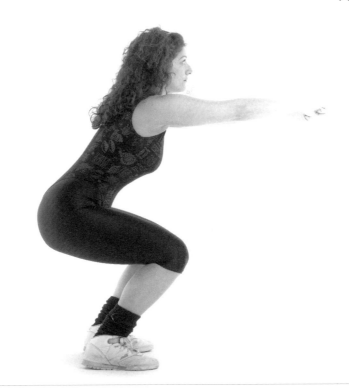

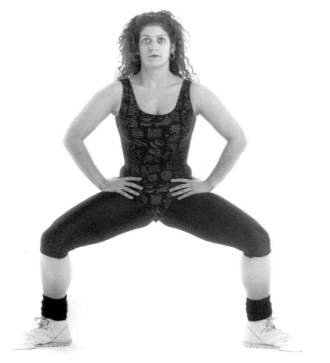

8. *Wide Stance Squats*

Starting Position:
Stand, feet shoulder width apart, knees soft, hands on your hips. Squat down.

Movement: 1. Move your feet out a half again. You will find that they will turn out in this position because of the distance of the stance. This isn't a problem as long as the knees point over the toes during the motion.

2. Squat up and down (the motion is slightly shorter than a normal squat). As with all squats, don't squat past the knees.

Reps: 25 for everyone.

THURSDAY

9. *Short Squats*

Before starting this one, you will probably have to shake out your legs a bit due to the build-up of lactic acid in the thighs. This is the elusive burn that everybody sought during the 80s. Forget it, remember 'any pain, no train'.

Movement: 1. Squat down, knees together, arms crossed in front at shoulder height (A).
2. Rise up half way to standing position (B), then squat again.
Reps: 25 for everyone.

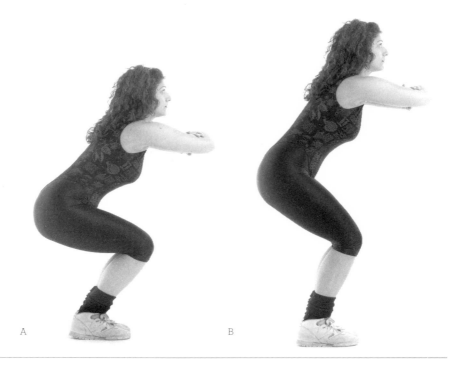

A   B

10. *Bent-Over Calf Raises*

You will need something to support yourself with this one, like the edge of a table or the back of a chair.
Starting Position: Bend over at the waist and rest your hands on your support, keeping your head in line with your shoulders and hands.
Place your feet shoulder width apart (A).

Movement: 1. Slowly lift the heels from the ground so that you are up on the toes (B). Hold for a few seconds and relax.
2. Start a pumping motion by lifting the heels from the ground and then back again without letting the heels touch the floor.
Reps: 20 for everyone.

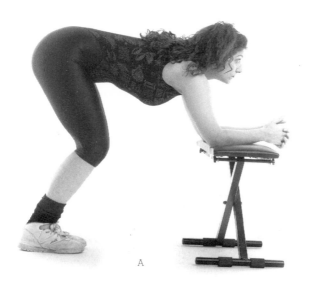

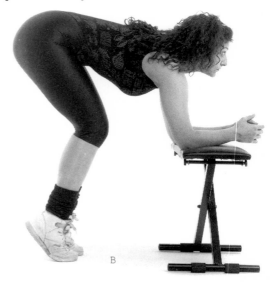

A   B

THURSDAY

11. *Straight Side Leg Raises*

Starting Position: Lie on your side, placing one hand under your head to support it and the other in front of the body to stabilise yourself. Bend your bottom leg back through 90° (A).

Movement: 1. Roll the top hip slightly forward and lift the top leg straight up, away from the bent bottom leg. Keep the hips and knees slightly rolled forward throughout the entire exercise (B).

2. When you lower the leg down, do so under control and don't rest it on the other at all for the whole set.

3. Change sides and repeat on yourself. (Don't forget to excuse yourself.)

Reps: Try 20 per leg.

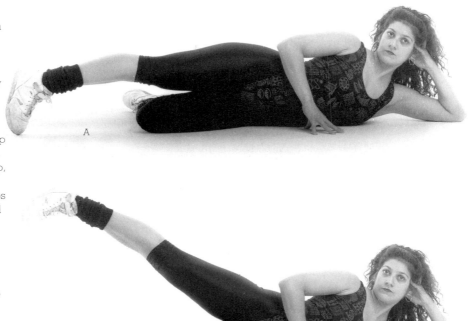

12. *Inner Thigh Raises*

Starting Position: Lie in the same position as the Straight Side Leg Raise, but with bottom leg straight. This time bring the top leg over the bottom leg and rest the foot on the floor. (The calf and thigh of the top leg should form a 90° angle.)

Movement: 1. Lift the bottom leg as far up as possible and then lower without touching the floor. Keep the hip, knee and foot facing forward throughout.

2. Change over legs and repeat.

Reps: Try 30–50 per leg as this is a faster exercise due to the small range of motion.

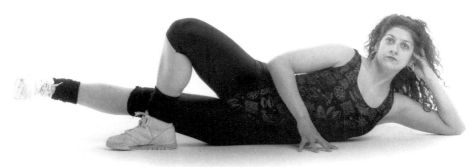

THURSDAY

13. *Dorsal Leg Raises*

Starting Position: On your stomach, head on your arms, and knees locked tight together.

Movement: 1. Curl one leg at a time to a 90° angle only. As you curl one leg press the other leg tight into the floor. At no stage try to stop the natural movement of the hips. If they start to raise slightly, let them.

2. Lower back to starting position under control. Concentrate on this one for best results.

Reps: 30–50 per leg.

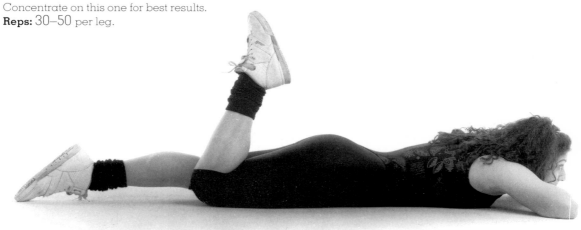

14. *Crunches*

Starting Position: Lie on your back, knees up, hip distance apart, ankles crossed.

Movement: 1. Frame the face with your hands and slowly lift your head and shoulders off the ground. Reach towards the knees.

2. Keep your back rounded throughout the exercise and try to keep your shoulder blades off the floor. Do not relax the muscles in your abdomen, and breathe regularly.

3. Return to starting position and continue.

Reps: 25.

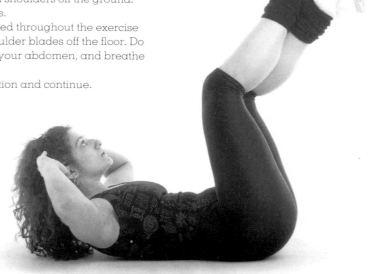

THURSDAY

15. *Diagonal Reaches*

Starting Position: Lie on your back, knees bent up, feet flat on the floor, hip distance apart. Hands behind or at the side of your head.
Movement: 1. Lift the head and upper back off the ground.
2. Reach across the body to the left knee with the right hand, then to the right knee with the left hand.
Reps: 20 per side.

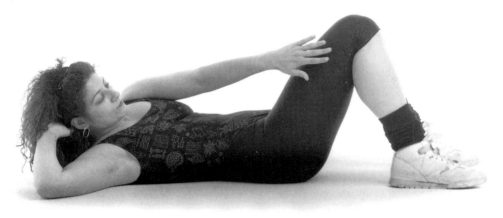

16. *Abdominal Pushes*

Starting Position: Lie on your back, knees bent up, feet flat on the floor, hip distance apart.
Movement: 1. Raise your left leg straight up towards the ceiling, and place your hands on either side of the extended leg.
2. As you lift the upper back and shoulders off the ground, push the hands forward and away from the knee.
Reps: 20 per side.

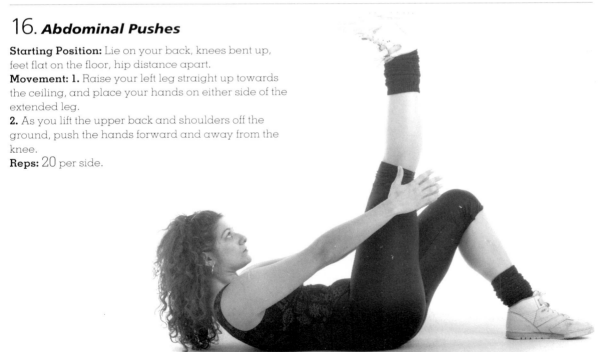

THURSDAY

17. *Side Reaches*

Starting Position: Lie on your back, knees bent up, feet flat on the floor, hip distance apart.
Movement: 1. Lift the shoulders and head up from the floor.
2. Put one hand by your head, and the other by your side. Reach alternately towards one foot then the other. The arm slides down the side of the body trying to touch the foot.
Reps: 20 per side.

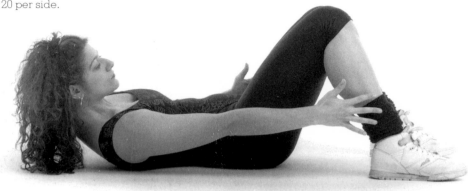

18. *Hyper-Extensions*

Starting Position: Lie on your stomach, place your hands on your bum cheeks, and cross your ankles behind you.
Movement: 1. Lift your upper body from the hips. All the pressure should be felt in stomach, hips and lower back.
2. Keep the position for 30 seconds, then release.
Reps: 25 for everyone.

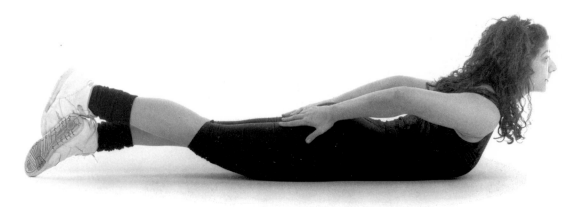

THURSDAY

19. *Bum Presses*

Starting position: Lie on one side and extend the legs. The hips should be slightly forward.

Movement: 1. Press the knee of the top leg over the other to the floor (A), and then return to the starting position.

2. When the top leg returns to the starting position the knee should point towards the ceiling (B).

Reps: Loads and loads, try 30 a side to start with.

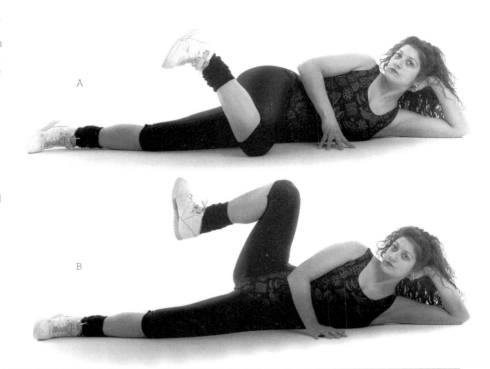

20. *Bum Lifts*

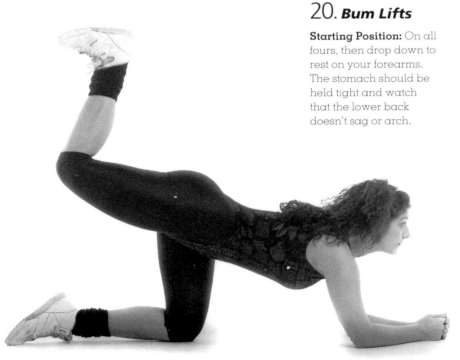

Starting Position: On all fours, then drop down to rest on your forearms. The stomach should be held tight and watch that the lower back doesn't sag or arch.

Movement: 1. Raise your right leg up and bend the knee, pointing the sole of the foot towards the ceiling (the angle of the knee and thigh should be 90°).

2. Push the leg up as far as possible without hyper-extending the lower back. The hips should stay square to the floor at all times.

3. Lower back to hip level under control. Again a very small motion so loads are expected.

Reps: 30–50 per leg.

THURSDAY

21. *Standing Bum Clenches and Pushes*

Starting Position: Stand up straight, knees together and slightly soft. Place your hands behind your head or on your hips.

Movement: 1. Clench your bum cheeks nice and tight.

2. Push to the right-hand side first, followed by the middle and then the left-hand side. The movement should be tight and small, a small thrusting motion.
It's all in the hips this one, so stay after class and practise.

Reps: Feel free to pump a enormous amount of these out. At least 30.

Now it's cool-down, time, then bang up the pulse to finish off. Take your pulse.

As this is a fairly sedate kind of workout, make sure that maximum effort is put into it. If you are feeling really lively after completing, try a few Burpees before cooling down and maybe a Stride Jump or 2,000.

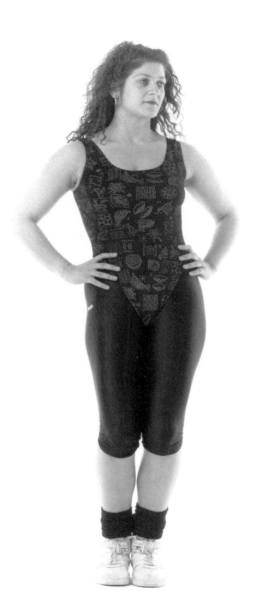

FRIDAY'S WORKOUT

THE BEST OF THE BEST

This is the ultimate in your workouts. It's tough, together and awesome. You've spent four days testing your physical and mental abilities to the limit, but you will have to be at your peak if you're going to win this one.

Friday's workout has all the best in it – muscular strength and endurance, an aerobic phase, flexibility, skill and coordination. Watch that pulse during this workout, as this is the workout to end all workouts.

Proceed through your warm-up and get ready to shake your thang.

The Fatbusting course, which should lose you up to 14 lb (6 kg), covers six weeks (30 days of work with 12 days rest). So you repeat the workouts each week.

However, as you work your way through the workouts, you will find that things get a lot easier. If so, try upping the tempo or increasing the number of reps you perform of each exercise, but as always, remember to maintain your pulse-training ranges (65–85% of 220 minus your age).

Let's have a quick technical look-see at the guidelines for conditioning related to exercise. There are three which must be part of any exercise programme – Overload, Progression and Specificity.

FRIDAY

Any type of exercise regime is governed by the above. Sticking to these three factors to the best you can, will give you the best gains in fitness as is possible for your body type, according to the genetic gifts given you by God.

Overload

Overload is considered to be the bee's knees of exercise conditioning. It's the number one aspect in achieving any great gains in health and fitness of any kind. Overload is incorporated into your fitness programme, by placing the body in a stressful position (but only nice stress) to bring about physiological and physical changes. Overloading doesn't need to be great, as long as it's constantly taxing the body. In other words, today's workout is next week's warm-up. Well, not quite, but a little should be added to each new workout for maximum results. Overload conditioning varies from person to person, and the way the body adopts to overloading relies heavily on three things:

1. The exercise programme you participate in.
2. The amount of exercise you do.
3. The intensity you exercise at.

Even though people have different responses to exercise (different strokes for different folks), nearly all people go through distinct stages on commencement of exercise. The first is quick gains in fitness and body shaping, particularly if you haven't had the pleasure of exercise before. At stage two you're still gaining, but at a slower rate with a lot more effort required. Usually the gains are far smaller, and this is a common time for drop out. Stage three is where we start levelling out, as we've nearly reached our genetic best. The returns for the time spent trying to achieve it will make you want to cut your throat, so make sure you achieve what you want in the first two stages of your fitness regime. Overload comes about by increasing the number of exercise sessions you perform and the length of time spent exercising. Do not increase the *intensity* until you are capable of completing your present exercise workload.

Progression

As demands of overloading are applied to the body, the body will adjust and adapt to the new stimulus. If progressive over-

FRIDAY

loading is achieved, the body will adapt wonderfully, but if the progression of the overload is too great, either from too much or too fast, it can lead to tiredness, injuries, soreness and, in the worst possible case, over-training, which can lead to you quitting exercise. Always remember, listen to your body at all costs. It's pretty good at telling you when enough's enough. It's probably taken you a good twenty years to get to the state you are in now, and it won't disappear overnight.

Specificity

'Train for what you need.' In other words, there's no point lifting every weight in the gym a million times to lose weight. Specificity is based on two major points:
1. What part of the body is being sorted out.
2. The part of health-related fitness being worked – ie. weight loss, heart and lung, flexibility etc.

FAT FACT

———— • ————

To keep the skin healthy, bump up the water intake. Loads of water flushes the system out. Start the morning with a mug of hot water and a dash of lemon to help clean out the digestive system. Eat plenty of fresh fruit and green vegetables, particularly broccoli, cabbage and sprouts.

———— • ————

Brilliant, so we know why we have to move on with our exercise programme from a technical point of view. From mine and your point of view, it would be pretty depressing and boring just doing the same few exercises every day and doing no more, no matter how fit and full of it we felt. Hence why we move on. Just because you're overweight, it doesn't make you a cripple. Go for it, dudes. See you in the next workout – on Monday again!

FRIDAY

1. Jumping Jacks

Starting Position: Stand tall, feet together, knees soft, hands by the sides.
Movement: 1. Jump both feet out to slightly past shoulder width. When you land make sure you bend your knees to absorb the impact.
2. As the feet land, the arms should be raised up to shoulder level height in the form of a cross.
3. Return back to starting position, hands at the sides.
Reps: 25 for everyone.

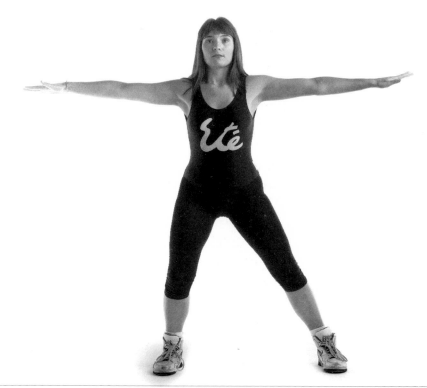

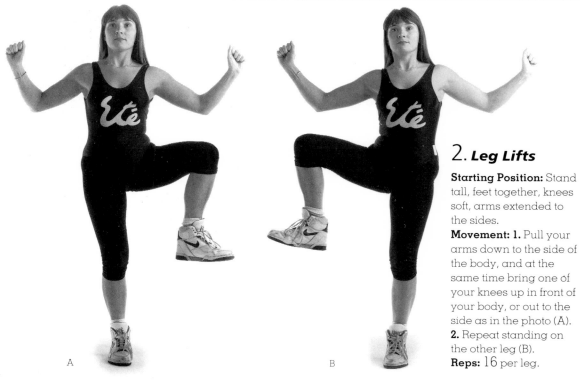

A

B

2. Leg Lifts

Starting Position: Stand tall, feet together, knees soft, arms extended to the sides.
Movement: 1. Pull your arms down to the side of the body, and at the same time bring one of your knees up in front of your body, or out to the side as in the photo (A).
2. Repeat standing on the other leg (B).
Reps: 16 per leg.

3. *Jogging on the Spot*

Stand feet together, stomach in. Jog on the spot, lifting your knees and pumping your arms. When you land, make sure you land on your heels then toes. Continue for 2–3 minutes to start with. Follow with some Marching on the Spot if you like.

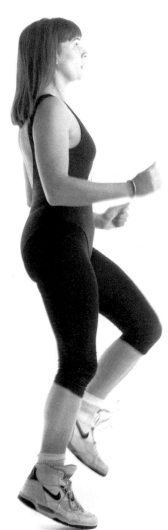

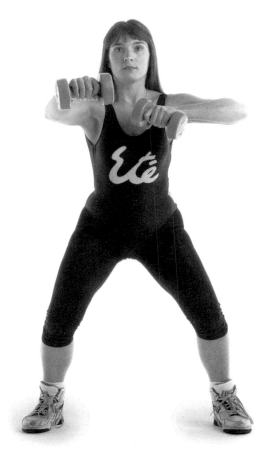

4. *Squat and Punch (with weights)*

Starting Position: Stand, feet shoulder width apart, knees soft. Hold the weights directly out in front of you at shoulder level height, with the knuckles facing the ceiling.

Movement: 1. Squat down to the Half-Squat position and hold.

2. Slowly extend the arms out in a punch motion, one at a time. Make sure you don't lock out the elbows during the punches. Keep the head upright and breathe regularly.

Reps: 20 per side.

FRIDAY

5. *Half Press-Ups*

Starting Position: Put the weights down and get down into a Half Press-Up position, on all fours. Straighten the back in a line from shoulders to knees, and keep the head up. Cross the ankles behind you (A).

Movement: Lower your nose to the floor, pivoting from the knees. Special attention should be paid to keeping the back straight as it will tend to sag (B). Again, don't lock out the elbows. And watch the hand placement.

Reps: 20 for everyone.

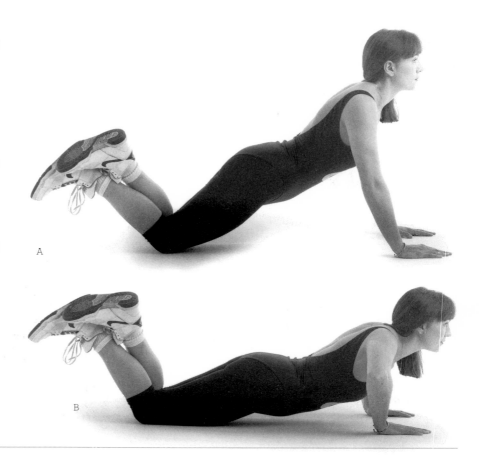

A

B

6. *Single-Legged Squat Thrusts*

Starting Position: Kneel down on the floor on all fours. Place the right leg straight out behind and tuck the left leg under the chest. Try and keep your head above the heart line (i.e. look straight ahead.)

Movement: 1. With a thrusting motion, change the legs, making sure the feet make contact with the floor. Keep the bottom down and the back straight throughout the motion.

2. Pay particular attention to hand placement throughout the exercise. The hands should be facing forward, elbows slightly soft and shoulder width apart. Under no circumstances, should the back sag during the exercise. The body should be tight and compact.

Reps: 10 per leg.

7. *Bench Dips*

Starting Position: Sit on a bench or chair. Place your hands facing forward on the edge of the bench or chair, shoulder width apart.

Movement: 1. Lift the body slightly away from the chair, feet in a box position to body, and the back as straight as possible (A).

2. Move the body down and up by bending the elbows out behind the body (B). Try not to raise the hips up at all during the movement, but use the arms always. Again remember not to lock out the elbows on the upward motion, and keep the back as straight as possible on the way down.

Reps: Try about 10.

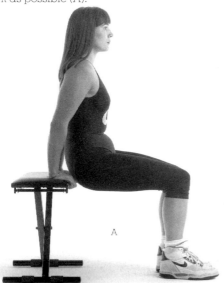
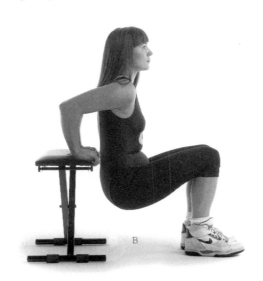

8. *Skip and Tuck Jumps*

Starting Position: Stand, feet together, knees soft.

Movement: 1. Squat down, keeping thighs parallel to the floor and put your hands under your knees (A).

2. Jump up, legs astride, arms reaching out the sides. Remember to keep your knees soft on landing (B).

3. Return to the Half-Squat position, and carry on.

Reps: 20 for everyone.

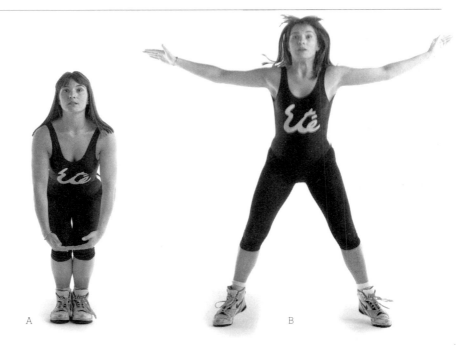

FRIDAY

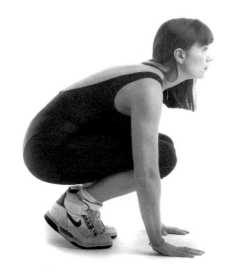

A

9. *Burpees*

Starting Position: Get down on all fours, then bring feet under hips (A).
Movement: 1. Thrust both legs out as in a Double Squat Thrust (B), bring them back under your hips, and then stand up straight (C).
2. Repeat the whole motion, and watch all the safety points of Single-Legged Squat Thrusts (on page 82).
Reps: A set of 10.

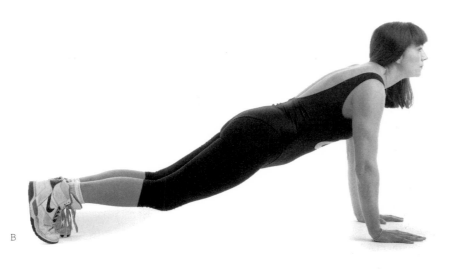

B

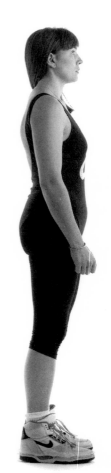

C

10. *Running on the Spot*

Start with marching on the spot, this time pumping the arms in the air, then break into a jog, followed by a run for 30 seconds. Make sure you land on your feet properly. Remember, if you can't whistle 'Dixie', give it a miss.

FRIDAY

11. *Stride Jumps*

Starting Position: Stand, feet together, knees soft, hands on hips (A).

Movement: 1. Keeping hands on hips and knees bent, jump both legs out and land shoulder width apart. Make sure when you land that your knees are kept soft, and feet are flat (B).

2. Return to starting position, and carry on.

Reps: 25 for everyone.

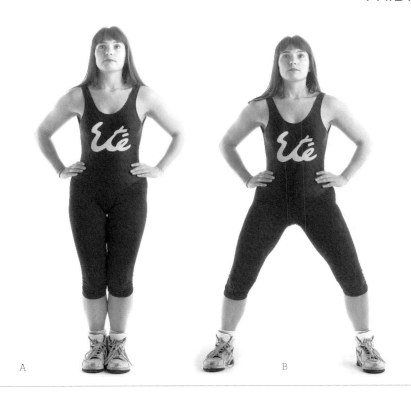

A   B

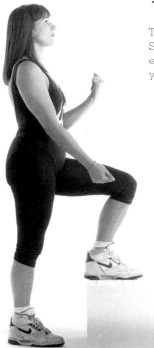

12. *Step-Ups*

This is exactly the same as the stepping you did in the Submaximal Test on page 41. Step up 15 times on each side. As you step, either keep your hands on your hips or curl them at the side.

FRIDAY

13. *Wall Crunches*

Starting Position: Lie down and place both feet against the wall, knees and lower legs bent at a 90° angle to the thighs. Press the spine into the floor and place the hands at the sides of the face as if framing a picture.

Movement: 1. Without moving the feet, slowly lift the shoulders off the ground, but taking care to keep the lower back pressed into the floor at all times. If your neck begins to ache at all during the exercise, place one hand under the neck and support it during the motion.
2. As you lift your upper body away from the floor, push against your stomach muscles for maximum feeling.
Reps: 30 for everyone.

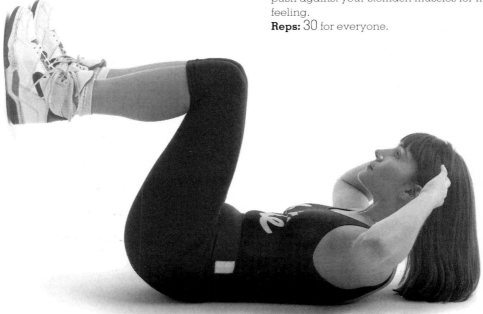

Proceed straight on to the cool-down flexibility work after completing your circuit. As it's Friday, and you've had a long week, you might be feeling like you've been to hell and back. It's probably just the sheer amount of work you've completed this week. Don't panic, but as you progress through the rest of your course, watch out for the signs of overtraining or exercise burnout.
When you overwork your body with *too much* exercise, you run the risk of this. You keep asking the muscles to deliver power and endurance without giving them the rest they need to replenish their energy stores. The symptoms include fatigue, boredom or depression, a change in appetite, insomnia or over-sleeping. If you end the week feeling shagged out and drained, you're probably doing too much. Your body is telling you to relax, rest and rejuvenate. Listen to the message and arrange your exercise schedule to allow for extra relaxation. If you persistently ignore the body's signals, or are unable to change your exercise schedule, you will suffer. Rest is the answer. Don't be a slave to the burn.

AT A GLANCE GUIDE

THE WARM-UP

1. *Walking around the Room*
2. *Jigging on the Spot*
3. *Shoulder Rolls* ×8
4. *Head Tilts and Chin Forward* ×8
5. *Short Squats* ×15/20/25
6. *Marching on the Spot* ×15/20/25
7. *Traffic Signal Squats* ×2
8. *Side-Stepping Arm Scissors* ×24
9. *Four Bent Knee Lift* ×4
10. *Diagonal Pumps* ×16 per side
11. *Grapevine* ×8 per side
12. *Side Lifts* ×16 per side
13. *Ankle Warm-Up* ×8 per foot
14. *Standing Quad Stretch*
15. *Inner Thigh Stretch*
16. *Spinal Compression Relief* ×4 per side
17. *Lower Back Stretch*
18. *Lunge*
19. *Hamstring Stretch*
20. *Second Pulse Raiser*

THE COOL-DOWN

1. *Back of the Arm*
2. *Chest Stretch*
3. *Neck Stretch*
4. *Upright Hamstring Stretch*
5. *Calf Stretch*
6. *Seated Inner Thigh Stretch*
7. *Outer Thigh Stretch*
8. *Hip and Back*
9. *Lower Back Stretch*
10. *Standing Shoulder Shrugs* ×20

AT A GLANCE GUIDE

MONDAY

1. **Free–Standing Squats** ×15/20/25

2. **Knee Lifts** ×8 per leg

3. **Stride Jumps** ×15/20/25

4. **Step Side Star Jumps** ×20 per side

5. **Marching on the Spot** ×16

6. **High-Impact Star Jumps** ×15/20/25

7. **Grapevine** ×16 per side

8. **Box Press-Ups** ×15

9. **Bench Dips** ×8

10. **Half Press-Ups** ×8

11. **Alternate Bicep Curls (with weights)** ×20 per side

12. **Alternate Shoulder Press (with weights)** ×20 per side

13. **Tricep Kickbacks (with weights)** ×15/20/25

14. **Single-Legged Squat Thrusts** ×10 per side

15. **Crunches** ×15/20/25

16. **Double Squat Thrusts** ×15/20/25

17. **Burpees** ×10

18. **Hyper-Extensions** ×15/20/25

19. **Jogging on the Spot**

TUESDAY

1. **Half Squat and Press** ×15/20/25

2. **Flying Laterals** ×15/20/25

3. **Standing Calf Raises with a Press** ×30

4. **Half Squats** ×15/20/25

5. **Stationary Lunges** ×15/20/25

6. **Side Lunges** ×15

7. **Pre-Ski** ×20

8. **Alternate Shoulder Press** ×15 per side

9. **Lateral Raises** ×15/20/25

10. **Alt Bicep and Head Curls** ×20 per arm

11. **Squat and Punch plus Half Press-Ups** ×20

12. **Tricep Chair Kickbacks** ×20

13. **Bench Dips** ×15

14. **Chest Flys** ×20

15. **Round the World with a Burpee** ×5/10/15

16. **Burpees with a Circle** ×5/10/15

17. **Marching on the Spot with Various Weights**

AT A GLANCE GUIDE

WEDNESDAY

1. **Reverse Crunches** ×20

2. **Diagonal Reaches** ×20 per side

3. **Side Reaches** ×15 per side

4. **Tight Crunches** ×15

5. **Pelvic Tilt with Bum Squeezes** ×10

6. **Hyper-Extensions** ×20

7. **Single-Legged Squat Thrusts**
×20 per leg

8. **Double Squat Thrusts** ×15

9. **Hyper-Extensions** ×20

10. **Floor Back Stretch**

11. **Crunch and Extend the Legs** ×10

12. **Abdominal Pushes** ×15 per side

13. **Jack Knives** ×15 per side

14. **Burpees** ×15

15. **Stride Jumps** ×25

16. **Standing Side Bends** ×20 per side

17. **Half Press-Ups** ×15

18. **Short Ab Curls** ×20

19. **Torso Stretch**

THURSDAY

1. **Free-Standing Squats** ×15/20/25

2. **Squat and Reach** ×15/20/25

3. **Forward Lunges** ×15 per side

4. **Tuck Jumps** ×25

5. **Stationary Lunges** ×16 per leg

6. **Skip and Tuck Jumps** ×25

7. **Pre-Ski** ×25

8. **Wide Stance Squats** ×25

9. **Short Squats** ×25

10. **Bent-Over Calf Raises** ×20

11. **Straight Side Leg Raises** ×20 per leg

12. **Inner Thigh Raises** ×30–50 per leg

13. **Dorsal Leg Raises** ×30–50 per leg

14. **Crunches** ×25

15. **Diagonal Reaches** ×20 per side

16. **Abdominal Pushes** ×20 per side

17. **Side Reaches** ×20 per side

18. **Hyper-Extensions** ×25

19. **Bum Presses** ×30 per side

20. **Bum Lifts** ×30–50 per leg

21. **Standing Bum Clenches
and Pushes** ×30

AT A GLANCE GUIDE

FRIDAY

*1. **Jumping Jacks** ×25*

*2. **Leg Lifts** ×16 per leg*

*3. **Jogging on the Spot***

*4. **Squat and Punch (with weights)** ×20 per side*

*5. **Half Press-Ups** ×20*

*6. **Single-Legged Squat Thrusts** ×10 per leg*

*7. **Bench Dips** ×10*

*8. **Skip and Tuck Jumps** ×20*

*9. **Burpees** ×10*

*10. **Running on the Spot***

*11. **Stride Jumps** ×25*

*12. **Step-Ups** ×15 per side*

*13. **Wall Crunches** ×30*

THE FATBUSTERS EATING PLAN

I've decided to deviate slightly from the rest of the book and touch briefly on dieting, and what I consider a good eating plan. This is due to the influx of wonder diets cum exercise programmes which have been hitting the pages of the magazines in time for the summer season. And once again the invasion is being launched from across the Atlantic. (I personally thought that the American invasion stopped with World War Two, but maybe all those GI babies are sleeper agents planted by the CIA, to confuse the public.) In recent years, we've seen the crumbling of the monarchy with the endorsement of an exercise and diet programme (yet to be proved to be effective), that in my humble opinion, comes straight out of Disneyland. The tabloids are always suggesting we slim for sex and follow celebrity diets. I guess this means that sex is out for the overweight, and all those rumours about plastic surgery and liposuction in the celebrity pack are untrue. The hip and lip diet is also with us, but the only pounds that you'll shed will be the ones from your pockets. (However, at least I think it's colour-coordinated.)

You've probably read about them all, no doubt tried them and possibly even had some success with a few. I decided to strike a blow for freedom, justice and the British way with a safe and proven eating plan to tailor to your own lifestyle, without too much messing around. What you're about to read is common sense, easy to adjust to and maintain, and, most important of all, if used in conjunction with your Fatbusters exercise regime, you will once and for all lose weight, Amen.

Eating in Restaurants

- Give takeaways a miss, but particularly avoid Indian and Chinese.
- In French and Italian Restaurants you can eat something like this:

Starter

Salad or crudités. Ask for the dressing to be separate, and forget to put it on, or try lemon juice or natural yoghurt.

Consommés and vegetable soups, especially those which are clear or tomato-based, not cream-based.

Beware of eating bread and butter when you are hungry before the first course arrives.

Main course

- Steamed or grilled fish without butter: Dover sole, rainbow trout, salmon steak.
- Grilled chicken (no skin), chicken kebabs, grilled liver or kidney.

With salad (without dressing, try lemon juice) or steamed vegetables (ask for them without butter).

Leave the potatoes alone because they are bound to be buttered or sautéed.
- Plate of pasta, with a tomato- or fish-based sauce. No cream- or butter-based sauces, ask specifically.

Dessert

Try fresh fruit, as it is generally available in restaurants.

In the Pub or Wine Bar

Most pubs and wine bars nowadays have Spritzers available. These are a mixture of white wine and Perrier or soda water.

- Drink slowly, so you don't get caught up in the drinks round buying.

- Try to only have one when other people have two.
- In the pub you can have a bottle or can of low-calorie low-alcohol lager. If you know the names of these beforehand, it is no different from asking for an unusual German lager, so nobody needs to know. Again drink slowly.
- If another drink is pushed on you, have a mineral water with ice and lemon or a tomato or other fruit juice.

The Eating Plan

The following eating plan is a seven-day programme that allows you one day off when you can have anything you like for your main meal. Decide which day that will be (most people choose Sunday) and call it Day 7. Make it the same day every week. You can start your programme whenever you want – just work out which day's menu you are on and start.

To get the best results from your eating programme:

- Follow the diet recommendations: don't skip meals or swap them around.
- Use no oil or salt for cooking, or on your food. Never fry, grill instead.
- Use herbs, spices or lemon juice to flavour your food, not sauces.
- Eat no sugar – use sweeteners or, better still, give it up for good.
- Always use skimmed milk in tea, coffee etc.
- Prepare your own lunchtime sandwich at home to take to work.
- Use only wholemeal bread, never white or 'brown'.
- Cut out all butter – use only low-fat spreads.
- Drink plenty of water, preferably bottled mineral water.
- Replace alcohol with sparkling mineral water with ice and a twist of lemon.

Weekdays 1–6

Breakfast   Sugar-free breakfast cereal with skimmed milk.

Mid-Morning Snack   1 piece of fruit (banana, apple, peach, pear, orange, nectarine, melon etc.)

Lunch   1 wholegrain sandwich or bap, or 1 baked potato with filling. No butter or margarine, use low-calorie polyunsaturated diet spread. No mayonnaise, oil or dressing.

Choice of fillings (one only) includes beef, chicken, turkey, hard cheese, egg, cottage cheese, tuna, smoked salmon, crab, prawn, salad, banana etc.

Mid-Afternoon Snack   1 piece of fruit.

Evening Meal   Large salad with low-calorie oil-free dressing or large selection of vegetables (steamed, quick grilled or raw)

with either 3–4 oz (75 g–100 g) grilled fish, grilled beef, grilled skinless chicken or turkey, hard cheese, cottage cheese, tuna, crab, prawns, smoked salmon, or 1–2 boiled or poached eggs.

Dessert   1 piece of fruit.

Evening Snack or Nibble   1 tablespoonful mixed nuts, without salt or chocolate/yoghurt coating.

Day 7

Breakfast   Sugar-free breakfast cereal with skimmed milk.

Mid-Morning Snack   1 piece of fruit

Lunch   This is your day off – have anything you want.

Mid-Afternoon Snack   1 piece of fruit.

Evening Meal   Large salad with low-calorie dressing with 3–4 oz (75–100 g) of meat, fish, chicken etc, or large fresh fruit salad, with no cream or syrup.

So as you have probably gathered, there are three very simple steps to eating well.

● Cut out all fats (within reason).
● Cut out all sugars.
● And watch the booze, it's the killer.

FAT FACT

————●————

It's one of the great injustices of time. As you get older, you tend to decrease your activities but your eating habits tend to stay the same. The rule of thumb to prevent this ailment is to cut your calorie intake by approximately 3% every 10 years from the age of 25. So by the time it's retirement age (65), it should be approximately 10% lower than when you were 25. Sad but true!

————●————

The Real Story: After Fatbusters

'I got up this morning, gazed into the mirror and realised I am thin again. How many mornings have I done this now? Not many, but the few that I have have been worth a lifetime. Pick up the morning rag still to have my optical senses assaulted by skinny little darlings selling every magic potion and cure available to modern man, but now I don't care because I look a thousand times better than the girl ever will. Now all I have to worry about is my gym and class membership and that's only once a year. The 90s has brought an era of peace and contentment, large curves and non-obsessive exercise behaviour. This still seems to be a problem because I'm still expected to be a certain size to be socially acceptable, but it's changing slowly – a bit like the 7.15 to Fenchurch Street, it's a-coming. I guess I really don't care that much, because I can run, jump and fight better than your dad can any day.

These days I'm not a brainwashed reader of the tripe that they pump down my throat any more, because now I'm an 'educated' fitness person. Between you and me, though, I sometimes fall victim to the occasional wonder cure, but then again I'm human like the rest of you. I still lose a pound here and there, but it's generally weekly now. Most of the classes are still not the kind of thing that suits me because they're full of scantily-clad birds paying homage to the gods of 'self obsession'. But there now seems to be a few more classes emerging for the common folk. Thank goodness for things like Fatbusters. But you know, the funny thing is, after a class I still crawl out and eat another chocolate bar . . . '

FATBUSTERS *on video.*

THE ORIGINAL
FATBUSTERS™

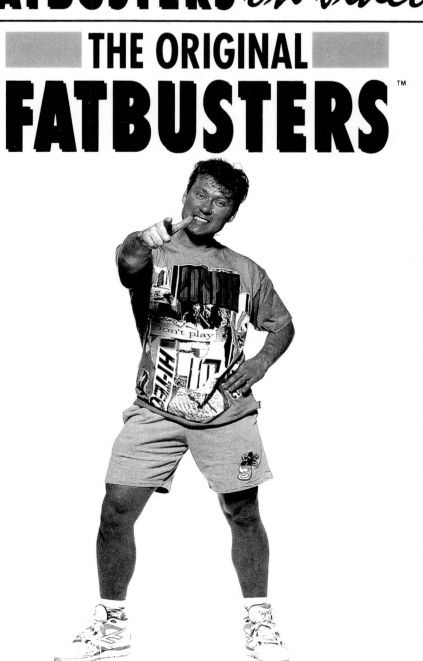

WITH JAMIE ADDICOAT-FITNESS
INSTRUCTOR TO THE STARS

WONDERLAND
FITNESS